Dr. Borko B. Djordjevic, M.D., Ph.D., F.I.C.S.
Dr. Dragan Cvetkovic

HAZARDS, NEGLIGENCE AND LIABILITY IN PLASTIC SURGERY

Handbook

Belgrade, 2022

Authors
Dr. Borko B. Djordjevic, M.D., Ph.D., F.I.C.S.
dr Dragan Cvetkovic

Publisher
„TIMELESS BEAUTY"
dnevna bolnica za plasticnu i rekonstruktivnu hirurgiju -
BEOGRAD

Consulting Editor
Prof. dr Milan Zarkovic, redovni profesor
Kriminalisticko-policijski univerzitet Beograd

Language Editor
Aleksandra Vitas

Technical editing and design by
„TIPOGRAFIK PLUS" - BEOGRAD

Printed by
„TIPOGRAFIK PLUS" - BEOGRAD

Circulation:
1000

Published by Quipper Prints
875 North Michigan Avenue,
John Hancock Center,
31st Floor,Chicago, IL 60611
www.quipperprints.com

ISBN (paperback): 978-1-77839-105-7
eISBN: 978-1-77839-106-4

Hazards, Negligence and Liability in Plastic Surgery - Handbook

Authors:

Dr. Barko B. Djordjevic, M.D., Ph.D., F.I.C.S.
(Chapters 1, 2, 3, 4, 5, 6, 7, 8)
Dr.Dragan Cvetkovic (Chapters 9,10,11)

Contents

REVIEW EXCERPTS

Prof. Milan Zarkovic, PhD

Authors of this Handbook hand to the users of health care services, health care professionals and all interested readers the text on a highly significant topic: hazards, negligence and liability in plastic surgery.

Nowadays, physicians, health care workers and citizens, being the users of health care services, know a lot, but there are still some patients and health care workers who are insufficiently informed and unready for the complex system such as health care within which, inter alia, numerous and diverse legal and ethical norms intertwine. Although the higher standard of the protection of patients' rights is achieved by acknowledging and reaching the active role of a patient in making adequate decisions concerning his or her health, medical quackery as a markedly retrograde and detrimental phenomenon is still present in contemporary practice.

On the way to coming closer to the soc1et1es of higher medical standards, with the developed network of various levels of social organization, which is characterized by disciplined respecting of rights which belong to medical workers as well as to the users of health care services, this Handbook may be of multiple benefits to both.

The selected matter is presented clearly and very precisely, with the assumed differences among the readers being taking into account, but with the emphasis on details which, at academic level, bring substantial and useful information of importance in recognizing, understanding and applying the principle of protection of rights of medical workers and the rights of patients in the health care systems in the US and Serbia, which is a sufficient reason for the best recommendation to the interested readers.

The Handbook comprehensibly presents the fact that despite the significant results achieved in the area of health care as well as the reforms in the legal framework which regulates the health care issues, the need for risk management is still essential. Through the review of the cases from practice, primarily in the US, the readers learn that there are still negative outcomes of the treatment and in rendering other health care services. Concurrently, the authors point to the significance of the implementation of the risk management plan with the aim of preventing cases of malpractice. The analysis of the cases from practice makes it clearly known to the readers that acting in accordance with the set standards, protocols, procedures can reduce the risk from a malpractice claim/complaint to a great extent. The Handbook makes it possible for the readers to learn about the potential health care risks and to better understand the legal basis of rights and obligations of patients and health care workers and the available mechanisms for exercising those rights and obligations.

The text implies that patients, as potential plaintiffs, agree that the prevention of malpractice is preferable to a lawsuit. In that regard, the authors pose the question whether it is possible to synchronize and control hundreds of variables which make the jigsaw puzzle of medical responsibility.

The authors of this interesting Handbook also show in a systematic, exhaustive and comprehensive manner the wide range of actions which may be undertaken in the context of criminal-law and criminal protection of human health in the Republic of Serbia. The special emphasis is placed on the criminal offenses regarding the protection of people from various acts (action or inaction) which relate to medical treatment and rendering other medical services, which may be done by both physicians and other health care workers (criminal offense of medical malpractice pursuant to Article 251 of the Criminal Code and failure to provide medical assistance pursuant to Article 253 of the Criminal Code) as well as by persons who engage in medical treatment or render other medical services, without appropriate professional qualifications, i.e. a university degree in medicine or dentistry, a diploma of secondary education in medicine etc. (the criminal offense of quackery and unlicensed practice of pharmacy pursuant to Article 254 of the Criminal Code). Following the analysis of the criminal-law protection of human health in general, with the special emphasis on the criminal offenses of medical malpractice, failure to provide medical assistance and quackery and unlicensed practice of pharmacy, the criminal aspect of acting with a view to preventing and suppressing medical quackery as a particularly dangerous phenomenon is shown.

One of the ways of bringing the Handbook closer to the readers are the examples from medical practice and the examples from judicial practice started for the infringement of patients' rights, including litigation for damages for injury caused as a result of medical malpractice. Thus, another goal of this Handbook has been achieved: giving the reader illustratively and gradually, step-by-step, the insight into the subject matter of risks a physician and other medical workers are faced with as well as patients in the area of health care and pointing to different outcomes in resolving proceedings and legal disputes primarily present in the US.

The content of the publication reflects the intention of the author, consistently implemented, to introduce the reader gradually and thoroughly to the subject matter. Thus, the Handbook may be a useful tool for the protection of rights in the area of health care. It has been elaborated in such a way as to the serve the need of physicians who wish to have a well grounded overview to risk management techniques with a view to reducing the frequency of claims/complaints for malpractice and thus indirectly and additionally ensure the quality within the health care system. This is a Handbook which will equally arouse the interest of medical workers and patients, health care and public health professionals, lawyers as well as of all the readers who wish to learn about potential risks in the area of health care and better understand the legal basis of rights and obligations of patients and health care workers and available mechanisms for effecting those rights and obligations.

The readers are recommended paying a special attention to this Handbook, all the more so for the fact that the topic of "man's health and rights in the area of health care" deserves detailed looking into and implementation for its special importance.

Generous sharing of personal experience in the selected area of exploration, which in case of prof. Barko Dordevic is linked to decades-long work in the field of plastic surgery in the United States of America and other developed countries of the contemporary world, will undoubtedly be an additional incentive to improving the measures and actions of prevention of occurrence of detrimental consequences in plastic surgery in our region. This will be especially done through raising the awareness of responsibility for assumed obligations and their fulfillment *Lege artis* by the care provider, of the risks which inevitably come with their work, but also of the necessity of additional caution of patients in choosing the person they will place their trust in and surrender to for performing plastic surgery procedures, and then of the possibilities of claiming rights to damages in case of negligence and injury caused.

It is evident that the Handbook is the product of the mutual cooperation of devoted people from medical and legal practice. The idea has stemmed from years-long practical experience of the author and his genuine care for the protection of human health. There are many other individuals whose ideas, acts and decisions have found place in this high-quality publication by author's selection, who also deserve praise.

PREFACE

The Handbook Hazards, Negligence and Liability in Plastic Surgery is intended for physicians, users of health care services, lawyers as well as readers who are interested in this important, but insufficiently discussed topic. The Handbook is designed in such a way that it can be a helpful reference tool in case of the infringement of rights in the area of health care. It has been elaborated in such a way as to meet the needs of physicians who wish to have a well established overview of risk management techniques which are effective in the contemporary surroundings.

The Handbook can be used within the program of continuing education of physicians, health care professionals, public health managers, employees of the health care organizations and institutions, lawyers who represent the users of medical services, i.e. patients, while it can also be useful to all the reader who wish to learn about the potential risks in the area of health care and better understand legal basis and obligations of patients and health care workers and available instruments for exercising those rights and obligations.

Human health is one of those values of the social community which (inter alia) are protected by criminal law. The right to health is at the same time one of the basic and most important human rights, which as such is guaranteed by both international-law documents and the Constitution as the most important domestic legal act at national level, while the protection of rights to health and health care is ensured by various branches of law. In that sense, the state is expected to ensure the health of people by incriminating all acts which endanger the health as well as by imposing criminal sanctions for those who engage in such acts.

The primary task of medicine is the protection of life and health, i.e. enabling the best quality treatment and the prolongation of the very life, respecting all achievements in contemporary medicine. Providing health care of people is based on the principles of accessibility, equity, continuity, efficiency etc. Why is the subject of health care so widespread? Many experts agree that the key issues are availability, affordability and quality of health care. Good quality health care is available, but critics make accusations of unacceptable prices. And price go up: many authors predict that the sum of money the society expends on health care will sharply increase in the course of the several following years. The components of costs do not only include the direct cost of providing health care (cost of work, capital costs of construction and equipment etc.), but also indirect costs which arise from hidden charges built in other fees. That includes the costs of lawsuits and defense as well as other factors in relation to liability.

The cost of lawsuit for malpractice expressed in money is as important as the psychological toll on both patients and physicians. Each physician who has been sued will confirm the enormous emotional strain which accompanies negotiations, defense or settlement. The same goes for patient-plaintiff ("Each patient is a potential plaintiff."): the process of seeking a lawyer, re-living the events which led to the suit and exposing details from their private lives to strangers is stressful and distressing.

All these worries are reasonable and all of them have implications for professional liability. Doctors who are unable to spend enough time with their patients believe that they are deprived of both the relationship and information. Managed decisions of health care institutions affect the patient outcomes and they will increase the liability of a doctor when the outcome is unfavorable. And when doctors are compelled to provide care to patients in an unsatisfactory environment, this can have a negative effect on patient care.

The result of the reforms implemented both in the field of health care and legal system, i.e. in the area of legal acts which regulate the issue of human health care is that the need for risk management has changed to a great extent, but it has not disappeared. There are still negative outcomes; lawyers continue to accept lawsuits for malpractice with the fee for work proportionate to success; and cases of actual malpractice continue to occur. For that reason, physicians have to take steps towards the implementation of the risk management plan so as to prevent cases of medical malpractice. Accurate records of treatment must be kept, a patient must be fully informed and he or she must have an active role in the medical treatment process. Acting in accordance with the adopted protocols, procedures and instructions will to great extent affect the reduction of the risk from a lawsuit/charges for medical malpractice.

And patients - plaintiffs agree that prevention and avoidance are preferable to a lawsuit. But is it possible in our complex society to control hundreds of variables which make a jigsaw puzzle of medical liability?

In the contemporary age, quackery is considered to be socially unacceptable and harmful phenomenon, and the activities of state authorities are directed towards suppressing this phenomenon. Thus, quackery is defined as a criminal offense in the national legislation of a large number of countries. quack doctors are persons who engage in medical treatments or render other medical services without having adequate qualifications and in that way they directly jeopardize people's lives, while in doing that, in most number of cases, they make illegal gain, which constitutes a criminal offense. The consequences of quackery may be extremely serious, especially with people of poorer health condition. With them, a certain infection may bring about a generalized systemic infection, and even sepsis. A disfigured face, injuries to the nerves, burnt skin and various deformations are some of the complications which may be experienced by persons who tend to subject to aesthetic corrections in flats and various salons where persons without adequate qualifications, i.e. quasi-experts work. Quack doctors inflict damage which is hard to repair, and, frequently, the damage inflicted is permanent.

Quackery has never been absolutely exterminated, i.e. there are sporadic cases in which certain individuals show more trust towards quack doctors than to real doctors. Nowadays, in our everyday lives, we often encounter examples of individuals addressing the very quack doctors for treatment, which can be confirmed by media reports on substantial expansion of quackery.

The criminal offense of quackery and unlicensed practice of pharmacy is stipulated in Article 254 of the Criminal Code of the Republic of Serbia, within the group of criminal offenses against the human health. This criminal offense is directed against human health, considered through the context of criminal-law and criminal aspect. Apart from criminal-law and criminal analysis of the criminal offense in subject, reference is made to the basic characteristics of the health care system in the Republic of Serbia.

"Risk management" is one approach in reducing the frequency and gravity of lawsuits for medical malpractice. Risk management practice involves recognizing schemes or acts within practice in subject (those which affect the filing of a lawsuit or prosecution), and then their removal or controlling so that the possibility of filing a lawsuit for medical malpractice would be reduced. Creation of medical records, making patients' appointments, issuing of prescriptions and communication with patients represent just a few of the customary activities which may have an effect on the possibility or the course of a lawsuit.

The goals of this Handbook are to provide assistance and be a significant tool in:

recognizing key elements and leading causes of lawsuits/ complaints for negligence and medical malpractice in traditional environments and in managed care environments.

determining the ways in which problematic relationships with patients may be resolved in both a traditional setting and a managed care setting.

risk control in doctor's office.

recognizing the risks related to managed care plans.

making decision on the most suitable ways of documenting a medical service and care provided to the patient.

recognizing risks related to quackery and other incriminating acts against human health.

Apart from the clearly defined educational goals, the content of this Handbook also intend to heighten the awareness of patients/ users of medical service of the importance of checking a potential medical service provider, a doctor or an institution before being subjected to any aesthetic procedure, treatment etc. This Handbook represents the starting point, but not the final answer for research and health care practice improvement. We hope this text will attract the attention of medical doctors, many health care professional as well as the user of medical services.

The text largely relies on the practice in the United States, considering the rich years-long experience prof. Dordevic has gained while working in all fields of reconstructive plastic surgery in the US. Being one of the leading plastic surgeons in the US, he won fame operating on the celebrities and public figures in the world of cinema, sports, music and politics as well as show business.

1. THE BASICS OF MEDICAL MALPRACTICE

Although some patients may perceive that malpractice has occurred when there is a poor or unexpected outcome, physicians know that's not true. A bad outcome, in and of itself, does not warrant a claim of malpractice. In fact, a physician's act, error or omission need not warrant a claim of malpractice, as long as the act, error or omission was reasonable under the circumstances.

The Four Elements of Malpractice

For our purposes, medical malpractice may be defined as any deviation from the accepted medical standard of care that causes injury to a patient.[1] To prove that malpractice took place, the plaintiff should be able to prove by a preponderance of the credible evidence four elements: duty, breach of duty, causation, and damages. If any one of these four is not proven, there should be no judgment of medical malpractice. On the other hand, the defense must negate only one element in order to prevail.

Duty

Physicians do not have a legal duty to treat anyone who walks into the office. In order for a legal duty to exist, there must exist a doctor-patient relationship. This relationship is usually established when the patient retains the doctor; but in some circumstances the relationship can be established by a third party, including a partner or a colleague with whom you consult. And, increasingly in this era of managed care, a doctor-patient relationship can be established by an HMO or network to which you belong.

---

1 *Malpractice: Don't be a target.* Louisiana Medical Insurance Company, 1990.

Consults and Referrals

To avoid inhibiting the free exchange of knowledge between physicians, the courts have generally held that informal consultations do not create a doctor-patient relationship. This doctrine was formulated in the landmark 1973 California decision, Rainier v. Grossman. Morton I. Grossman, a professor of gastroenterology, had lectured several physicians at their hospital, then offered to review their own cases with them. One doctor presented the x-rays and medical history of Mary M. Rainier, who suffered from ulcerative colitis. Without examining the patient, Grossman advised surgery, which was subsequently performed. Rainier sued, alleging that the surgery had been unnecessary, and listed Grossman as a codefendant. An appeals court upheld summary judgment in Grossman's favor, noting that he had no duty to the patient because he had no direct contact with her and no control over the treating physicians.[2]

Direct patient contact is not, however, a prerequisite for establishing a duty, as witnessed by the 1982 Illinois decision, Davis v. Weiskopf. Plastic surgeon Jerome S. Weiskopf examined Mr. Davis in a hospital emergency department. An x-ray of Davis' knee revealed a likely malignant neoplasm, so Weiskopf referred Davis to orthopedist Philip D. Brooks but didn't tell the patient why. Davis failed to show for any of the three appointments he scheduled and Brooks refused to reschedule him. Davis subsequently died of cancer, and his estate sued Weiskopf and Brooks. A lower court granted summary judgment to Brooks, but an appeals court reversed, ruling that a doctor-patient relationship began when Brooks accepted the referral and scheduled the patient. The court also said "a letter to plaintiff advising him of his condition and that he should consult with another physician without delay might well have been sufficient" to discharge his duty to the patient.[3]

---

2 *Rainer vs. Grossman*, 3 I Cal App. 3ʳᵈ 539, Ct. Of App. 2ⁿᵈ Dist, 11ᵗʰ April 1973.
3 *Davis v. Weiskopf*, III. App. 64, 439 N.E. 2ⁿᵈ 60, I 08 III., App. 3ʳᵈ 505 (1982).

Another potential point of liability is the informal consultation.[4] Has a colleague ever asked you for your opinion about the condition of a patient whom you've never examined? These "curbside consults" can, under certain circumstances, be construed as establishing a doctor-patient relationship. Courts have traditionally held that informal consultations between physicians do not create a doctor-patient relationship, and have usually granted summary judgment in favor of the non-treating physician. However, the definition of the doctor-patient relationship has broadened in recent years and it's often difficult to tell whether you owe a duty of care or not. For example, if both you and the treating physician are under contract with the patient's managed care plan, you may be just as involved as if you'd examined the patient yourself. Even the other doctor's mistaken impression that you had agreed to a formal consult might create a relationship exposing you to liability.

Fortunately, you can reduce your own liability without alienating your colleagues by making sure that all parties clearly understand whether you're giving gratuitous advice or assuming an active role in patient care. Begin by having your attorney review contracts you are considering with managed care plans to determine your responsibilities to plan members who are not currently your patients. Likewise, if you serve as an on-call doctor with your hospital emergency department, learn the limits of your responsibilities whenever you give advice to the treating physician.

Next, keep notes of your consultations, no matter how informal. This doesn't mean opening a chart - just a simple note of who you talked to, what you were told, what advice you gave; and the date. Don't record or even ask the patient's name unless you're making an appointment to examine him - the less you know of specific identities the better. State clearly whether you agreed to examine the patient, and document when no referral is requested. Such notes will not only limit your liability, but can actually improve the quality of your advice by helping you to focus your thoughts and by making it easier to keep track of what information has and has not passed between you and the other doctor. Once the attorneys step in, your colleague may feel sure you were provided with more information than you actually received.

---

4 Cynthia Shea Goosen,. *How a Curbside Consult Can Land You In Court.* MedRisk Monitor, July 1994. at I.

Finally, discussions of whether you will examine the patient yourself should never be left open ended. Either commit yourself ("I will see him in the morning") or make it clear that you have not committed ("Call me back if you want me to examine him.") Don't leave it open by saying "If he's not better in the morning I'll take a look at him." Such vagueness may very well be a liability later.

Walk-In Patients

Unless you hold yourself out as willing to treat walk-in emergencies, you may have no obligation to treat someone entering your office that is not already your patient. That was established by a Texas decision, Salas v. Gamboa. After delivery by a midwife, the newborn son of Roberto Salas developed breathing difficulties. A nearby hospital refused to treat the infant, so Salas took him to the office of family practitioner Jose Gamboa. There, a medical technician immediately asked Gamboa if he would care for the child. Gamboa refused, and instead referred them to a children's hospital. The baby died hours later, and Gamboa was sued. An appeals court upheld summary judgment for Gamboa, stating that, "a physician is not to be held liable for arbitrarily refusing to respond to a call of a person even urgently in need of medical or surgical assistance provided that the relation of physician and patient does not exist at the time. "[5]

Note: In the Salas case at no time did the doctor or his staff agree to offer care. Actions by the staff may be binding on the doctor, and even the receptionist's offer to work the baby into the schedule might well have established a duty to treat.

Contract Arrangements

A doctor-patient relationship may exist any time a physician renders services on the patient's behalf under contract. In Peterson v. St. Chad Hospital, a 1990 Minnesota appellate decision, LeeRoy Peterson sued for damages caused by unnecessary chemotherapy for a lung nodule that was first diagnosed as small cell carcinoma but later proved to be a bronchial carcinoid tumor. Among the defendants was R.A. Murray, the pathologist who prepared the initial diagnostic report. The court denied summary judgment because Murray had a contractual relationship with Peterson's

---

5 *Salas vs Gamboa*, 760 S.W. 2nd 838 (Tex.App.-San Antonio)

treating physician, had performed services under that contract with the expressed or implied consent of the patient, and therefore had established a doctor-patient relationship with Peterson.[6]

Managed health care plans may also create a doctor-patient relationship any time a physician employed by the plan consults in the care of an enrollee, as shown in Hand v. Tavern. San Antonio resident Lewis L. Hand, a member of the Humana Health Care Plan, presented to the emergency department of a Humana Hospital complaining of a three-day headache. Hand explained that he had a history of hypertension and his father had died of a ruptured aneurysm. An emergency physician on duty attempted to stabilize Hand with medication. Hand's condition remained unstable, so the treating physician telephoned internist Robert Tavera, who was in charge of screening HHCP admissions, for permission to hospitalize. Tavera declined authorization, advising instead that Hand be treated as an outpatient. Hand went home and suffered a stroke a few hours later. He sued the hospital and Tavera for negligence. The hospital settled and a lower court gave summary judgment to Tavera on the basis that no doctor-patient relationship, because Hand and Tavera had never met.

On appeal, the higher court opted to scrutinize the contracts binding Tavera and Hand with Humana. One clause that caught the court's attention stated, in part, that:

Physician agrees to provide enrollees with medical services which are within the normal scope o physician's medical practice. These services shall be made available to enrollees without discrimination and in the same manner as provided to physician's other patients.

In a 1993 ruling, the court concluded that the wording of the contracts "brought Hand and Tavera together just as surely as though they had met directly and entered into a doctor-patient relationship. Thus, summary judgment in the doctor's favor was reversed, allowing Hand to pursue a malpractice claim against Tavera.[7]

---

6 *Peterson vs. St. Cloud Hosp.,* 460 .W. 2nd 635 (Minn. App. 1990)
7 *Hand vs Tavera* 864 S. W. 2d 678 (Tex.App. - San Antonio 1993)

5

The deciding factor in this case was the specific wording of the doctor's contract with the plan. Likewise, hospital medical staff bylaws can also act like a contract, to establish a duty between doctor and patient. If you are on call for the ER, there is a duty to the patients who will be seen under that arrangement. However, if you are volunteering to take call, rather than doing so because it's "your tum," the circumstances may be different. In the 1991 Fought v. Soke decision, a Texas appeals court ruled that a physician who had voluntarily served on-call was not under contract, and therefore could refuse to treat anyone who was not already his patient. However, the court made clear that, had the doctor been under contract to serve on-call, or had served as a condition of maintaining staff privileges, such obligations might well have created doctor-patient relationships.[8]

Insurance and Employer Physicals

Generally, performing an examination at the request of a third party does not establish a doctor-patient relationship. This opinion was expressed in the 1977 Johnston v. Sibley decision, in which an appeals court ruled that a doctor's "duty to use a professional standard of care in making the examination and preparing the report runs only to the party requesting it."[9]

That doctrine was cited in the 1992 Wilson v. Winsett decision. Gerela Standifer had applied for disability benefits, and was referred to internist E. Merrill Winsett for evaluation. Winsett found a hilar mass on x-ray, which was recorded in his report to the referring agency. Standifer, however, did not learn of the mass until four months later, when another physician discovered it and diagnosed bronchogenic carcinoma. Standifer died the following year and her estate sued Winsett for failure to report his findings to the woman or her doctor. An appeals court upheld summary judgment for the doctor on the basis that Winsett's only duty was to the agency.[10]

---

8 *Fough1 v. Solce*, 821 S. W. 2nd 218 (Tex.App. - Houston, 1991, writ denied)
9 *Johnston v Sibley*, 558 S.W.2nd 135, ref. n.r.e.
10 *Wilson v. Winsell*, 828 S.W. 2nd 308, 309.

A critical element in the Wilson decision, however, was that Standifer had not requested information from Winsett about the examination. Compare that with an otherwise similar 1977 decision, Caldwell v. Overton, involving a woman who was examined to verify her eligibility for worker's compensation. In this case, the examinee had inquired about the doctor's findings-and had copies of the report sent to her personal physician and to her lawyer. The appeals court ruled that a doctor-patient relationship had been established when the person being examined inquired about and received medical information from the examining physician.[11]

Defense attorneys advise that any of the following actions may, for legal purposes, initiate a doctor-patient relationship:

Billing the patient for any service.

Making any contact with patients of another physician for whom you are providing coverage.

Accepting a referral from another physician, even if the patient fails to show.

Scheduling a patient for an appointment or agreeing to see a walk-in, even when done by your staff.

Discussing your medical findings with or providing records to someone you have examined on behalf of an insurance company or other third party.

You may be liable for the actions of your partner who takes call for you in a group practice. Similarly, if you take call for your partners and through that arrangement you see one of their patients who later sues, the charges will probably be filed against you as well as your partner. This liability may arise even if you are a solo practitioner sharing space and services with other solo practitioners because the courts may hold that your loose affiliation with the others is actually a partnership.[12]

11 *Caldwell vs Overton*, 554 S.W.2nd 832
12 *Ask the Experts*. Insurance Corporation, of American Malpractice Report, May 1992.

Informal consultations are not the only way you may unknowingly establish patient relationships. If you treat a patient as a "good Samaritan" yet later bill the patient for your services, you probably will be held to have established a relationship. Although good Samaritan laws vary among the states, most provide immunity from civil damages to physicians who provide their services for free to those who need emergency care. Certain conditions apply and may vary from state to state. In Texas, for example, the Good Samaritan statute does not protect individuals who regularly administer care within a hospital emergency room, nor does it protect the patient's admitting physician or associated treating physician of the patient.[13] If you render emergency care and do not bill the patient, the Good Samaritan statutes will protect you within the guidelines of the law. If you do bill the patient, you probably won't be protected. These guidelines seem clear-cut but become less well defined for emergency care rendered within the physician's office. A recent case was decided in favor of the plaintiff who alleged negligence on the part of her physician who rendered emergency care for an episode, which took place in the doctor's office. The physician did not bill the patient for the emergency care, but did bill her for the other services rendered as part of the examination which brought her to the office in the first place. That bill prompted the court to dismiss the Good Samaritan defense.

As noted above, your receptionist or office staff can also establish duty. If a patient needs prompt attention and is told that you will see him "shortly" or at a specific time in the future, a duty has been established because the patient may then relax and remain in your office where his condition may deteriorate, rather than attempting to find a quicker source of care.[14] *Make sure that your office staff is familiar with procedures for handling patients who claim to be in distress and that you are promptly notified of their presence in your office.*

---

13 H. A. Thompson, *Volunteer Liabilily.* Tex Med, July 1991 at 58
14 *M.P.Demos, The ABCs of Risk Management for Today's Praclicing Physician,* 77 J. Fla. Med. Assoc. 37 (1990).

Breach of Duty (Negligence)

Once duty has been established, a plaintiff must demonstrate that the physician failed to render the required standard of care, traditionally defined as that level of care a reasonably prudent physician would provide under similar circumstances.15 Failure to do so results in the breach of duty, which constitutes negligence.

The traditional definition has undergone some modification in recent years. Instead of adhering to recognition of community or local standards, there is increasing emphasis on a national standard of care. A recent decision by the Indiana Court of Appeals held that "a physician is under a duty to use that degree of care and skill which is expected of a reasonably competent practitioner in the same class to which he belongs, acting in the same or similar circumstances." Under this standard, advances in the profession, availability of facilities, specialization or general practice, proximity of specialists and special facilities, together with all other relevant considerations, are to be taken into account.16

Nor is it sufficient to claim that ordinary or customary practice is "good practice." As one court said, "It is entirely possible ... that what is the usual or customary procedure might itself be negligence."17

Who-establishes the standard of care? In court, expert witnesses for each side will endeavor to testify convincingly, as detailed in section five of this book. Standards set by specialty societies also are being promulgated as the "standard of care." More and more, though, defendant physicians will be facing allegations that they failed to comply with practice parameterA' that have been developed for certain specialties and conditions.

---

15 David M. Hamey, Medical Malpractice, Charlottesville VA, The Michie Company, 1993., p. 506
16 Centman v. Cobb, 581 N.E. 2nd 1286 (Ind. App. 1991)
17 lundhal v. Rockford Memorial Hospital Ass 'n, 93 Ill. App. 2nd 461, 235 .E. 2nd 674 (1968).

Practice Parameters

Practice parameters (also known as practice guidelines, practice policies and clinical pathways) are strategies for patient management which, in most cases, are designed to assist - not govern - your clinical decision-making. Parameters include protocols for pain management, performance of caesarean sections, and testing for allergens responsible for immunologically mediated diseases.[18] Thousands of practice parameters exist today and they vary in their purpose, depth, and development methodology.

Where do parameters come from? They are developed by specialty societies, the federal and state governments, academic medical centers, hospitals, and other sources. They usually have their source in the medical literature and hospital studies, which then are adapted to local practice.

Many physicians fear that practice parameters will increase their exposure to allegations of negligence, especially in cases where the physician may not be following the parameters for a certain course of treatment. The AMA suggests that such fears are unfounded because most parameters will not become absolute standards.[19] During the course of malpractice litigation, the standard of care is likely to be determined on a case-by-case basis, not on the basis of nationally publicized practice parameters.

Practice parameters will, however, become an important part of the pool of information to which plaintiffs, attorneys, defendants, and various experts refer during the course of litigation. And some states are adopting parameters for other purposes. For example, Florida's Health Care and Insurance Reform Act mandates that the agency overseeing health care administration "develop, endorse, implement and evaluate scientifically sound, clinically relevant practice parameters." The purpose is "to reduce unwarranted variation in the delivery of medical treatment, improve the quality of medical care, and promote the appropriate utilization of health care services."[20]

---

18 *Practice paramelers: a physician's guide to their legal implications,* Chicago, AMA, 1990.
19 Id., p.4
20 *Florida 's grand experiment addresses praclice paramelers.* J Florida Med Assoc, Vol. 81, No. 3, March 1994.,pp. 184-189

In Maine, a pilot project places practice parameters squarely at the center of malpractice defense. Physicians who take part in this project and use specific adopted parameters in their practice will be considered to have provided the standard of care, even if there is a poor outcome. Therefore, the parameters provide an affirmative defense in a medical liability claim.[21]

Practice parameters are going to serve other purposes as well. The government is establishing parameters as part of its effort to hold down health care costs. By establishing "standard" ways to address medical problems like management of herniated lumber discs, the parameters may lessen the need for certain tests or therapy. Physicians are divided on the use of parameters for cost containment. Some believe guidelines are overdue and that parameters will improve the quality of care by reducing unnecessary variations in diagnostic and treatment methods. Others believe they are an unnecessary intrusion into the practice of medicine and fear that parameters may actually reduce quality by discouraging innovation.[22]

Consultants and the Standard of Care

As a physician, the standard of care may require you to render care in accordance with the diagnosis and treatment recommended by consultants you call in on a case. Whether you agree or disagree with the consultant, you may be liable for any damages incurred by the patient.[23]

In some cases a physician may be held liable for the negligence of another physician to whom patients are referred. Courts have ruled that a referring physician must use "reasonable care" when referring to another doctor. If the plaintiff can show that the physician "knew or should have known" that treatment by the referred physician posed an unacceptable risk, the referring physician may be held liable for the negligence of the other.

To protect yourself against allegations of negligent referral defense attorneys advise the following:

Avoid relationships with other physicians which could be characterized as employer-employee.

---

21 Press release from the Main Board of Registration in Medicine, December 20, 1991
22 *Guidelines spread, bur how much impact will they have?* Med Econ, July 12, 1993., pp. 66-89
23 Demos, MP. *The ABCs of risk management for today's practicing physician.* J f'la Med Assoc, January 1990., p. 36

Do not bill patients for other physicians' services.

Let the patient know that each physician is an independent contractor and that no physician is responsible for the care or treatment rendered by any other physician.

If you practice m a partnership, be aware of your partners' competencies.

If problems with quality of care arise, take steps to correct them.

Be aware that if you refer the patient to a colleague at night or on weekends, someone who is on call for the person to whom you actually referred the patient may see the patient. Consider finding out who is on call for your referral physicians.

If you observe substandard care being rendered by a physician to whom you referred the patient and you are still providing concurrent care, don't ignore the substandard care. You could be held liable if the plaintiff is able to prove that you knew about it but did nothing to correct the problem.

Causation

Next, it must be proven that the breach of duty was the cause of the patient's injury - in other words, that-the physician's failure to adhere to the standard of care caused a situation or event that resulted in harm to the patient.

The jury can find that a physician failed to conform to the standard of care, yet decide that this failure was not the cause of injury. In Neal v. Welker, the patient fell and sought treatment at a hospital emergency room. The defendant physician failed to discover a skull fracture and, after prescribing aspirin, sent the patient home to bed. The patient suffered severe brain damage and eventually died. The defense prevailed, however, despite the defendant's negligence, by showing that proper treatment (i.e., timely diagnosis and treatment of the skull fracture) would have made no difference in outcome. [24]

---

24 *Neal v Welker.* 426 S. W. 2nd 476 (Ky. App. 1968).

In another court case that serves as an example, the plaintiff alleged that a hospital was negligent in failing to diagnose hypoglycemia in a newborn during the first six hours of life and that the alleged negligence was the cause of the child's mental retardation. Although the plaintiffs expert made a convincing case for negligence, the defense presented evidence, which suggested that the child's injuries were caused in utero, rather than by anything that happened during or after birth. The jury found for the defense and, although many jurors believed the hospital was negligent, they also believed that negligence had nothing to do with the child's injuries.[25]

Damages

The final element that the plaintiff must prove is damages, which may be defined as the sum of money a court or jury awards as compensation for a tort or breach of contract.[26] There are different types of damages. *Monetary* or *economic damages* include money that the plaintiff must spend in order to rectify or manage the injury allegedly caused by the physician. Included would be the cost of items, which are readily quantifiable: repeated surgeries, round-the-clock nursing care, institutionalization, the cost of household help, special equipment, clothes, etc. Monetary damages also include money lost from the plaintiff's inability to work. *Non-economic damages* include compensation for the plaintiff and/or the plaintiff's family for alleged pain and suffering or mental anguish. Other types of non-economic damage are alleged loss of consortium and interference with the ability to enjoy life. *Punitive* or *exemplary damages* are money sought for the purpose of punishing the defendant for an intentional tort or gross negligence or for the purpose of deterring others from taking a similar approach to patient management.

---

25 *Mattie McDonald et. Al. Vs. Bolnice Sr Joseph,* Civil Action No. 87/38564, filed in 152nd Judicial District Court, Harris County, Texas.
26 Campion FX. *Grand Rounds on Medical Malpracrice.* Chicago, American Medical Association, 1991., p. 351

In most cases the plaintiff must provide expert testimony, not only to show that the breach of duty caused injury, but also to quantify the past and probable future physical: effects of the injury and to detail the past and future medical and nursing expenses. The jury is permitted only to hear about damages that an expert will say are going to occur. In contrast, a jury would not be permitted to award damages for a negligent delay in the - diagnosis and treatment of breast cancer if the plaintiffs expert could only opine that the delay increased the patient's risk of dying from breast cancer by ten percent.

In most malpractice cases damages are based on obvious injuries -brain damage, death, loss of a limb, etc. These are the cases that most plaintiffs' attorneys are willing to accept because there is the greatest possibility of obtaining a large award from the jury and the corresponding contingency fees paid to plaintiffs' attorneys will be greater. However, the court system does not prohibit cases, which may carry lesser damages. A plaintiff may sue for any reason, and if the plaintiff can't find an attorney to take the case, the plaintiff may file on his own behalf. Such cases must still be defended, and since the cost of .defending even non-meritorious suits can reach tens of thousands of dollars, there is often an incentive for the physician and insurer to settle the case for a specific amount of damages.

Case Study #1

A patient in her mid-twenties visited the defendant ophthalmologist for a routine eye exam. Due to her young age a glaucoma test was not performed. She later was diagnosed with glaucoma and sued the defendants, alleging negligence in failing to perform the test.

The defense argued that the standard of care was to not administer the test to patients younger than 40 because the instance of glaucoma at younger ages was so rare.[27]

Which of the following statements do you think best describes the applicable standard of care in this case?

The defense should prevail because their actions were reasonable, customary and prudent, given the standard of care (go to #1 below).

---

27 *Helling vs Carey,* 83 Wash 2nd 514,519 P.2nd 981, 67 A L.R. 3rd I 75 (1974)

The plaintiff should prevail because all patients should be protected against glaucoma, regardless of their ages (go to #2 below).

Discussion

1 You said that the defense should prevail, based on the prevailing standard of care. That's what the original jury said too, and that verdict was upheld on appeal. The defendants introduced evidence that the incidence of glaucoma in patients under forty years of age was only one out of 25,000. The jury was instructed on rules regarding the standard of care, defined as a "duty to perform the degree of care and skill expected of the average practitioner acting in the same or similar circumstances." However, the state supreme court reversed, and returned the matter to trial court to determine damages. For the court's reasoning, see below.

#2 You said that the plaintiff should prevail because all patients should be protected against glaucoma, regardless of their ages. The jury and appeals court both found for the physician defendants, but the state supreme court reversed and returned the case to the trial court to determine damages.

Comment

In its opinion, the court went so far as to say that it was "the duty of the courts to say what is required to protect patients under the age of forty from the damaging results of glaucoma.: Seven facts were cited, including the facts that the test was well known, easy to perform, inexpensive and conclusive. Also mentioned was the fact that glaucoma could be treated if caught early, but irreversibly damaging if undetected.

This is an example of a case where the standard of care was found to be neither the local custom nor the national custom, but rather was based on what "should be" the custom.[28]

Case Study #2

A 45-year-old man saw the defendant family physician for a physical exam and treadmill test. He returned eight years later for a follow-up treadmill test and physical. Both times, results were normal. In the interim he also saw the defendant several times for earache, pneumonia arid a back problem.

---

28 For discussion see *Harney supra*, p 508-509.

Four years later the patient called the defendant, Dr. Parker, complaining of epigastric pain focused between the xyphoid and umbilicus. The defendant told the man to take Maalox and go to the hospital to pick up a prescription for Prilosec. Dr. Parker further instructed the patient that, if he was still experiencing pain, to go to the hospital ER and not leave until he had been examined.

The patient took the Maalox and picked up the prescription but did not go to the ER. He suffered an MI shortly thereafter and died. The survivors sued, alleging that additional stress testing should have been done between the first and second stress tests because of the family history of heart disease, of which Dr. Parker was aware. The plaintiffs also argued that the prescription for Prilosec was inappropriate and that a referral to the ER should have been made immediately.

Which of the following statements regarding negligence would be most likely to prevail in court?

The patient was negligent in failing to follow the physician's instructions to go to the ER (see #1 below).

The physician was negligent in failing to more closely monitor the patient's heart condition (see #2 below).

1 You said that the patient was negligent in failing to follow the physician's instructions. Although this is one those cases which could be argued either way, the defense argued that the patient was indeed negligent for several reasons. First, the patient had been advised to schedule repeat physicals and stress tests, but had not done so, a contention supported by the medical record. Second, the defense argued that the patient's complaints were consistent with epigastric problems and that if the patient had gone to the ER as directed he probably would have survived.

The jury found for the defense on the basis of the patient's own noncompliance.

#2 You said that the physician was negligent in failing to more closely monitor the patient's heart condition. That's what the plaintiffs said, alleging that the physician was negligent in attempting to diagnose over the phone. However, the defendant's testimony and medical records stated otherwise. In fact, the doctor had advised the patient to schedule physical examinations and stress tests, but the patient had not complied. That, coupled with the obvious non-compliance with the directive to go to the ER, was sufficient for the jury to find for the defense.

Comment

This case illustrates the importance of documenting non-compliance in the medical record, a point that will be examined in greater detail later in this book.

Case Study #3

A physician began treating a patient for severe abdominal pain in November 1997. Diagnosing Crohn's disease, he treated her for about three months and during that time he noted a sausage-shaped mass in her lower abdomen. However, he ordered no tests to determine its nature. In February 1998 the patient was diagnosed with terminal cancer which originated in her bowel. She died two months later and her family sued, claiming that she experienced unnecessary pain and suffering and died prematurely because of the misdiagnosis.[29]

Which of the following defenses will likely prevail in this case?

The physician was not negligent. Crohn's disease was a likely diagnosis, given the patient's history and condition (see #1 below).

The physician may have been negligent, but there was no causation. The missed diagnosis did not cause the patient's death (see #2 below).

Discussion

1 You said, that the best defense would be to argue that the physician was not negligent. The problem is with his own notes, which indicate he knew-there was a mass yet did nothing to investigate it. The standard of care would suggest that further testing be done to determine the nature of a "'sausage-shaped mass" in the lower abdomen. Therefore, the assertion that the doctor was not negligent would very likely fail.

#2 You said that the best defense would be based on the issue of causation. By asserting that the missed diagnosis did not cause the cancer or the patient's death, the defense would likely prevail.

---

29 Based on *Dowling v. Lopez*, 440 SE.2nd 205 (Ga. Ct. of App., Dec. 3, 1993; certiorari denied Feb. 22, 1994.)

In fact, that's what happened. The trial court entered summary judgment for the physician, noting that there was no evidence that the misdiagnosis was the proximate cause of the patient's death. There was no proof that the patient didn't have terminal cancer when the doctor first started treating her.

2. RELATIONSHIP ISSUES

Much of the previous chapter focused on the technical nature of the patient-physician relationship. However, the interpersonal side of the relationship is also a factor in medical liability risk management. Patient-physician relationships play an enormous part in the patient's decision to sue. Some studies suggest that as many as 63 percent of suits are based on communication issues: failure to keep the family informed; the patient's desire for revenge; or the perception that the physician or other members of the health care team were avoiding the family.[30] Other estimates go as high as 80 percent.

Not only is the relationship between patient and physician critical in malpractice avoidance, the relationship among physicians, nurses, therapists and other health care professionals can also play a role. Hickson et. al. discovered that one-third of plaintiffs sue because they are urged to do so by another member of the medical team.[31]

This section will examine the patient-physician relationship and the relationships between physicians and other medical team members as those relationships affect quality care and risk management.

Why Do Patients Sue?

Why do patients sue? We have surveyed nearly twelve thousand physicians on that very question, and consistently get the following responses:

Unrealistic expectations. Patients today expect perfection. They read, watch health segments on TV, and are well aware of the advances in modem medicine. When they have a medical problem, they expect that today's physician can solve it through a combination of medical science and technology. When there is a less-than-perfect outcome, patients may feel betrayed by the very system they expect to protect and heal them.

---

30 Hickson GB i drugi. *Factors that prompted families to file medical malpractice claims following perinatal injuries.* JAMA, 267: I 0, I 359/1363.
31 Ibid., p. 1359

Poor rapport and poor communication. As previously noted these factors play a i large part in the patient's decision to sue. Few patients will sue a doctor they like and trust because they don't want to damage that relationship. On the other hand, if the patient perceives that the doctor or his staff representatives are cold, uncaring, or rude the patient may be more inclined to sue if something goes wrong.

Greed. Money is seldom the primary factor influencing a patient's decision to sue but it is a complicating factor. Patients may read of the multi-million dollar awards made by juries to plaintiffs who were able to prove their cases in court to the jurors' satisfaction. Non-meritorious suits and the awards they generate also receive press and can further influence the patient's desire to sue.

Lawyers and our litigious society. The United States has more lawyers than any other country and almost three times as many lawyers per capita than Great Britain.[32] That may be one reason American malpractice claims run 30 to 40 times higher than Great Britain's. Another is the contingency fee. In many other countries the contingency fee is illegal but not in the United States. Why not? One reason is our prohibition against making the loser of a lawsuit pay the winner's legal expenses. In other countries which allow that practice, lawyers have good reason to take on a meritorious case even for a poor client. In our system, unless the client has independent sources of money, the only place for attorneys' and legal fees to come from is the recovery itself.[33]

Poor quality of care. There are two types of quality: quality in fact and quality in perception.[34] Both are important in risk management. If there is poor quality in fact, that means the patient is receiving care that is not up to standard. If there is poor quality in perception, the patient will believe he is receiving substandard care, even if that is not the case. Both can lead the patient toward an attorney's office.

Poor outcome. Unless the plaintiff can prove that the four elements of malpractice exist, a plaintiff's attorney will not take the case. Therefore, there must be a substantive reason for the patient to sue. "Poor outcome" is a precipitating factor.

---

32 Olson WK. *Can we ever hall America's lirigarion epidemic?* Med Economics, September 16, 1991., p.121
33 Ibid., p. 125
34 Townsend P. *Commit to quality.* New York, John Wiley&Sons, 1990, p. 4.

Failure to keep the family informed. Such things as not returning phone calls and letting family members know how their loved ones are doing can create hostility and a perception that you are rude and uncaring, and both conditions breed a propensity to sue.

Although this is by no means a comprehensive study of reasons patients sue, it is a composite list of the reasons most frequently given by physicians when asked why patients sue. It also matches reasons listed in other studies of malpractice.[35]

Patient-Physician-Staff Relationships

"Poor relationships with patients" and "poor communication" play a surprisingly large role in a patient's decision to sue. Of course, patients don't sue exclusively because their doctors don't communicate well; but if things go wrong during the course of treatment, or if there is an unexpected outcome, poor relationships make it much more inviting for the patient to get back at you by filing a suit. In fact, it has been stated that "the critical variable in the filing of a malpractice claim is neither clinical error nor iatrogenic injury: it is the patient or the patient's family."36 A noted plaintiff's attorney agrees, saying that many patients turn to lawyers when they feel they can't get information or believe the doctor is avoiding them or giving them the runaround. "A lot of patients who come in are confused or are getting conflicting information," says Jim Perdue. He tells doctors that the best way to avoid being involved in a lawsuit is to maintain good patient rapport.37

The same holds true for medical office staff. Patients will decide if receptionists, nurses, and other assistants are "good" largely by the way these staff interact with patients. A friendly, warm interpersonal environment will make it easy for the patient to believe that the quality of care is good, too.

---

35 Paxton H. *Why doctors get sued.* Med Econ, April 18, 1989., p. 44
36 Orlikoff JE i Vanagunas, AM. *Malpractice prevention and liability control for hospital.* Chicago, American Hospital Publishing, 1988., p. 113
37 *Risk management can ease liability woes.* Am Med ews, December I, 1990, p. 16

Communication plays another role as well. Patients tend to judge their doctors on social criteria, not clinical criteria. Clinical competence is assumed. Therefore, patients will decide if they like you the same way they decide if they like their friends and neighbors, and may decide to change doctors on the basis of your communication abilities. A recent survey shows that as many as 44 percent of patients have switched physicians recently because of the doctor's attitude or the attitude of his office staff.[38] Others haven't switched doctors, but mention that the thought has crossed their mind more than once. And, once the patient begins to feel that the doctor is uncaring, it is less likely the patient will share information or concerns that could be crucial to the diagnosis or treatment for fear of being rebuffed. Now the relationship really is in trouble, and the only one who has the ability to get it back on track is the doctor.

These tips, of course, have to do with "bedside manner." What is good bedside manner? Answers vary, but in general it's concerned with treating patients as human beings worthy of your time and attention. For many physicians that goes without saying. For some, however, it bears repeating. As risk manager Lin Tuthill puts it, "If you act like God you'll be expected to perform like God." And that's a sure invitation to a lawsuit.[39]

Remember, patients who like their doctors and medical office staff, and feel a strong sense of loyalty and friendship toward them, are much more inclined to resist the notion of suing, even if things do go wrong.[40]

---

38 Eisenberg H. *Patient Loyalty: you are doing something right.* Med Econ, Aprila 23, 1990, p. 50
39 Tuthill EL. *Documentation for medical staff* Tampa, Florida, 1994.
40 Gafner RS i Launey CL. *Techniques of reducing the frequency of medical-legal lawsuits using paracommunication and neurolinguistics.* Hjuston, Medical Risk Management Inc., 1989.

Common Patient Complaints

Among common complaints are the following:

"He interrupts me too often." In fact, some studies have shown that the average length of time a doctor allows a patient to speak before interrupting is only 18 seconds.[41] Why is it so common for physicians to interrupt? Most physicians are taught to keep patient interviews on track, and if they perceive that the patient is starting to ramble they interrupt to bring the conversation back on course. However, remember that patients, like most of us, are brought up to believe that it is not polite to interrupt, and they may well perceive the physician's interruption as rude, even if it is clinically necessary.

"She doesn't answer my questions." This is one of the most frequent factors cited in a patient's decision to file a suit. When the patient or family member has a question that isn't answered to their satisfaction, or if they feel ignored, they become anxious, then angry; and may think that the physician is ignoring them because there is something to hide. In such cases they may seek answers in the medical record, which often leads to outside evaluation by attorneys and hired experts - evaluation that can lead to litigation if the medical record suggests that care was questionable.

"The doctor talks down to me or talks over my head." Patients today are sophisticated consumers of medicine. A patient may resent a doctor who talks simplistically when the patient is able to understand more sophisticated explanations. The opposite is also true at times: "The doctor talks over my head." Terms that you explain once then use routinely can cause problems if the patient didn't understand your explanation. Consider the example of the patient with gall bladder disease who was facing surgery. Her surgeon stated that he would perform a laparoscopic cholesystectomy and proceeded to explain what was involved. During the explanation he referred repeatedly to a "lap choly." When he was finished he asked if the patient had any questions and she said timidly, "I don't understand where the dog comes in." The physician was quite surprised that she had interpreted his term "lap choly" to be a lap-sized collie.

---

41 *Medical science seeks a cure for doctors suffering from boorish bedside manner.* Wall Street Journal, March 17, 1992.,p.B-1

"She doesn't spend enough time with me." A sick patient is an anxious, nervous human being who longs for reassurance, or at least acknowledgment from the physician that efforts are being made to make things better. However, if the physician seems to give the patient only a cursory visit, or doesn't spend "enough" time, the patient will resent that. A recent study showed that the average physician spends less than five minutes with each patient during hospital rounds. Patients believe it's less; physicians believe it's more-but it's only about five minutes. Another study found that general practitioners spend less than seven minutes talking with the average patient during office visits. Although the doctor may be able to do everything that's needed during that time, the patient probably will feel shortchanged-especially he is presented with a bill for that visit that doesn't adequately reflect the perceived value of the amount of time spent with the doctor.

"The doctor; doesn't listen to me." This complaint underlies most others. If the patient's question is ignored or answered flippantly, or if the patient wants to hear about what's happening to him but the doctor doesn't stay long enough, the underlying perception may be that the physician is a poor listener.

A point to remember: many patients may complain to your staff instead of you. They may not want to "bother" you with what they think is a personal perception; or they fear that you will become angry if they bring up something negative.

Countering Complaints

The above are common patient complaints that can produce relationship problems if allowed to progress. In addition to posing risks, they can also affect the patient's perception of quality of care. Here are some tips to counter them.

Show that you're listening. Listening is often downplayed as a factor in communication; however, its role is critical to understanding and enhancing relationships.

Of the four traditional communication skills, we spend most of our time listening and the least amount of time reading and writing. However, the time spent learning how to do each is reversed. In school, we're taught reading and writing from the first grade up, but listening is seldom a part of our formal education. Why? Possible because there's tendency to equate "listening" with "hearing," but the two are very different. Listening takes effort, and there are definite factors which get in the way of effective listening. For example:

Thinking about what you will say next. This type of dysfunctional communication is called a duologue. When one person speaks it is very common for the listener to hear the first part of what is said, then start to formulate his response while the speaker is still talking. As a result the listener doesn't really hear the last part of what is said and may miss a critical part of the conversation.

Keying in on facts and details while ignoring the broader message. In medicine you must gather as much information as you can but it is easy to let facts get in the way of understanding the patient's overall message. This is a learned habit: our educational system encourages paying attention to facts and details by testing us on them as we go through school. As a result, when a patient says, "I first noticed these symptoms about two weeks ago; it was right after I got back from vacation," the physician may zero in on the fact ("two weeks ago") and overlook the part about the vacation. Doing so may make a difference if the vacation site or events may have played a part in the patient's symptoms.

Faking attention. With increased emphasis on good patient relations as both a practice management and risk management technique, most doctors today know the power of listening. Unfortunately, knowing what to do and doing it are often quite different. While the patient is talking many doctors may be guilty of reading the chart, making notes, or even thinking about what to say next. However, since they know they should be listening instead of doing these other things they may well "fake" attention, thus running the risk of missing an important piece of information or of alienating an astute patient.

Try active listening as both a diagnostic and quality improvement tool. Active listening is a technique that encourages the patient to talk and gives you valuable information you won't get by asking straight "yes" or "no" questions. Most listening is passive: the speaker talks and the listener just sits there. Active listening takes listening up a notch. The active listener takes part in the conversation, by periodically summarizing what the speaker says, searching for content, and not judging. Here's how it works:

Ask the patient an open-ended question, one that can't be answered "yes" or "no" and requires the patient to think before responding. When she responds, use nonverbal cues that show you are paying attention: nod, frown, raise an eyebrow, or demonstrate other "attending" behaviors. When the patient is through, paraphrase what she said by feeding it back to her, using your own words to summarize the meaning.

When you are actively listening, watch out for traps. It's easy to get caught up in what the patient is saying, or to judge or evaluate what she is saying, or to let your mind wander. Doing so will sabotage your active listening efforts and you will probably appear insincere to your patient. Active listening is appropriate for counseling situations but you may not want to use it during yes/no interactions, such as taking a history.

Spend quality time. As noted above, a major patient complaint is that the physician doesn't spend enough time with the patient. This complaint is rooted in perception, such as the perception that the patient doesn't get enough time and attention from the physician to justify the bill.

Physicians, on the other hand, must accommodate scheduled patients, emergency cases, hospital rounds, employee interactions, consultations with colleagues, and dozens of other activities. No wonder patients may perceive that you are in a hurry.

Solution: Maximize the quality of the time you spend with patients, without spending much more actual time. Here's how.

When you are conversing with the patient or family member, before or after the physical exam, sit down. Pull a chair up within easy conversational distance, and look at the patient while you're asking questions and getting answers. Physical contact is good, too, within reason. The act of taking the patient's pulse, or a reassuring hand on the shoulder, has dramatic impact on the patient's perception of you and the quality of your interaction.

If you take these simple steps your patient will have a different opinion about the quality of time you spend and even the amount of time you spend.

The Structure of Rapport

Rapport is the state produced by a close and sympathetic relationship. It's marked by agreement and harmony between and among its participants.

In patient relationships, rapport is the intuitive sense that the doctor and patient share fundamental things in common. There are different kinds of rapport.

Body rapport is a common way of moving, gesturing, and behaving.

Voice rapport is a similar way of using words, tone of voice, pitch, speed, and other vocal cues.

Content rapport is created by a sense of understanding, as indicated by actively listening and paraphrasing.

For the doctor, rapport is important not only in principle; it's also a critical ingredient in achieving quality in perception and in preventing medical liability claims. This is true for several reasons:

A patient who feels rapport with his or her doctor may be less likely to want to pursue a claim, even if one may be warranted.

A patient who has rapport with his or her doctor will be more likely to do what's necessary medically to carry out a course of treatment.

A doctor with good patient rapport will find it easier to talk with the patient about his or her treatment, and will discover that it's easier to obtain informed consent for those procedures requiring such consent. Patients who feel rapport with their physicians will likely perceive a higher standard of quality in your care.

Establishing rapport is easy when it's done subtly. It's a matter of reading nonverbal cues and responding appropriately.

Body Rapport

Body rapport is a similar way of moving, gesturing, and positioning one's body.

Consider Dr. Robbins, an animated and energetic family physician. She uses frequent gestures to illustrate the points she makes in conversation and moves quickly when she walks. She is quick to smile and laugh when appropriate, and is often called "a bundle of energy." Her new patient, Mr. James is quite different. He speaks slowly and walks much more slowly, not because of any physical problem but because he doesn't see the point of hurrying to get anywhere. He ponders what he says for some time before actually speaking, in sharp contrast to Dr. Robbins who speaks quickly and responds quickly when it is her turn to talk. People who talk with their hands drive him crazy.

After his first encounter with Dr. Robbins at the HMO clinic, Mr. James requested another doctor. His reason? "She makes me nervous by moving around so much." Dr. Robbins was relieved when he left, because she was feeling frustrated with his slowness to respond to her questions.

To create rapport with her patient, Dr. Robbins could have noted Mr. James' manner of speaking and moving and taken steps to mirror his behavior. Mirroring is a means of establishing body rapport and voice rapport. To mirror another person's behavior, observe what he does then, a few moments later, do something similar. If he crosses his legs, cross yours. If he leans forward and nods, do the same.

A key point: mirroring is not the same as aping. Don't copy the other person's behavior explicitly. Pace your actions so that the change in posture or gesture appears normal. This is important for two reasons: first, you don't want to give the appearance that you are copying every nuance; and second, you don't want to appear phony. By waiting a few moments to make your shifts you will appear much more normal.

What types of behavior can you minor to achieve rapport? Gestures, body orientation, posture, tone of voice, how fast you talk, choice of words-all are candidates for mirroring.

Mirroring is important because it creates the subtle impression of similarity with the other person. Remember, most people like themselves; and if you seem to be like them they will probably like you.

Another important point: Although mirroring is a powerful tool for achieving rapport, don't attempt it if you are uncomfortable or don't believe in the concept. One physician we know takes exception to the notion of mirroring, stating that physicians, "like heads of state or bishops, are trained in dignified ways of behaving" and to mirror patients would disrupt that dignity. Our position: like any other tool, if you don't feel comfortable with it, don't use it.

The Immediacy Principle

The immediacy principle states that people draw closer to people, things or situations they like, prefer, or feel comfortable with. They draw away from people, things or situations they're uneasy with or don't like.

Why is this important? By observing your patient's nonverbal behavior you can literally get a glimpse into his or her hidden feelings about you and your staff. The immediacy principle allows you to understand how people feel about you and others.

Advertisers know this. The phone company has been inviting us for years to "reach out and touch someone."

Immediacy can be literal, as when people physically draw closer to others or to things.

When you 're shopping for a gift for someone special, what do you do when you see something that interests you? You get closer so you can see it better. On the other hand, until you see something you like, you're careful to keep some distance between yourself and displays; to do otherwise might indicate to a salesperson some interest on your part that isn't real.

Immediacy can also be psychological, as when there is no physical closing of distance but other channels are used to signal the desire to approach (eye contact, response time, body orientation or gestures).

Immediacy is communicated through multiple channels:

Gestures (kinesics)

Use of space (proxemics)

Use of the eyes

Choice of-words

Environmental factors

Each of these channels is useful to the doctor m both creating immediacy and in reading immediacy in patients.

Gestures

Research indicates that one of the components of "warmth" is the noticeable use of gestures during interaction.[42] People who "talk with their hands" are usually rated as warmer and more friendly than are people who are very reserved in their use of gestures.

You're at a party telling one of your favorite stories. You find yourself gesturing to illustrate your point, and when you finish, discover that your audience has grown from one politely interested listener to half a dozen.

---

42 Gafner RS. Nonverbal cues ofwannth. Unpublished doctoral dissertation, University of Houston, 1976.

29

Sound reasonable? Your warmth and enthusiasm, as signaled through nonverbal cues, drew people closer to you.

Some people are naturally reserved. They don't use many gestures themselves and they don't like to be around people who do. If this describes you, try abbreviated gestures. No need to make wild arm swings when a small hand swing will do. For people who don't like to gesture, the power is the same. It's a nice compromise.

Use of Space

The way you use space in patient interaction is a powerful indicator of immediacy. Remember that people draw closer to people they like and feel comfortable with and pull away from people they dislike or feel ill at ease with.

Studies of how people use space in talking with others has produced some interesting observations. Hall draws four concentric circles in his analysis of the use of personal space.[43]

Most business interaction in America takes place within personal distance - from about 18 to 30 inches from each other. This holds true for most conversations, especially those in which only two people are involved.

If more than two people are talking, the "proper" space moves to the social sphere. At social distance (about 30 to 48 inches), you can still talk in a normal tone of voice.

At more than four feet, or public distance, you must raise your voice slightly (or greatly) to be heard. You wouldn't feel right having a personal or business conversation at this distance; public distance is for discourse and one-way interactions.

Physicians operate under different spatial parameters than most people. By definition, a physical examination requires that the doctor touch the patient. Thus a doctor routinely operates at intimate distance with the patient. It's necessary and expected; and under most circumstances the patient doesn't perceive that the doctor is "invading" personal space. But what effect does this have on perceived immediacy?

---

43 Hall E. *The hidden dimension.* New York, Doubleday Anchor, 1966.

The answer lies in what's "normal" and "expected" during routine interpersonal encounters. Routine encounters include business meetings (group or one-on-one); grocery shopping; talking to your spouse after a day's work; and other similar circumstances. For a physician-patient relationship, the physical examination, including prolonged touch, is also normal and routine. But once the examination is complete and the setting or environment changes (i.e., the encounter moves from the examination to discussion), then the parameters change. It's no longer normal or expected for the doctor to be touching the patient as before. Now, the unwritten rules regarding routine interpersonal encounters apply.

To be perceived as warm or immediate, the doctor in the office setting should demonstrate the same spatial or proxemic cues that are expected under other circumstances. For example:

The physician sits forward in her chair. Her hands are open and visible on top of her 3 desk. She leans forward, further closing the distance between herself and her patient. She looks directly at the patient at all times and, when the patient is talking takes care not to look away or down at her desk.

The nonverbal cues in this example are congruent with the physician's attempt to project an attitude of warmth and liking. Every cue that closes distance (leaning forward, direct eye contact, leaning the head forward, arms and hands forward to minimize distance) supports immediacy.

In contrast:

The doctor leans forward in his chair, writing notes in the patient's record. He doesn't look at the patient, either when he (the physician) is talking, or when the patient is talking to him.

Eye Contact

Eye contact is the psychological equivalent of direct touch. It establishes a powerful bond between two people. That's why it's so stressful to maintain direct eye contact for prolonged periods of time.

Have you ever been in a staring contest with a child? Who wins?

The kid will win every time. That's because children haven't been socialized the way adults have. The longer we've been around in society, the more we learn to behave and conform to societal expectations. One such expectation is that "nice people don't stare", because staring makes others uncomfortable. It's that psychological bond, the psychological intimacy that comes from direct eye contact.

Choice of Words

The words used in conversation are revealing. They communicate a sense of immediacy (or lack of immediacy) by revealing the speaker's attitude toward the subject of the conversation.

You ask your nurse to bring you specific records. She enters your office with records in hand, places them, on your desk, and says, "Here you go. "

You ask your nurse to bring you specific records. She enters your office with records in hand, places them on your desk, and says, "There they are. "

What's the difference?

In the first example, the nurse uses the word "here." She's associating herself with the records and probably with you.

In the second example, the nurse is placing subtle distance between herself and the records and your request for them.

Environmental Factors

Your office and other surroundings over which you have control send out signals about how you feel about yourself, your patients, and your relative status.

The office has a big desk, with two guest chairs in front of the desk. There's also a separate seating area with sofa and side chairs, clustered around a coffee table. Where would you sit to communicate greater immediacy with your patient?

Your guide in this exercise is the size and number of barriers, and actual or perceived distance, between you and the patient. If you sit behind your desk, that's one big barrier. If you lean back in your chair, putting more distance between you, that's another barrier. If you swivel so you're angled away from the patient, that's another.

Reversing those cues, you could lean forward, facing your patient directly. For even more immediacy, you could come out from behind your desk and sit in the guest chairs, angled so you're facing the patient. If it's going to be an extended conversation, the seating area would be a good place to go.

The key here is eliminating as many perceived barriers as you can, thereby increasing immediacy.

Nonverbal Leakage

You're running late with your scheduled appointments, and are due at the hospital for rounds in ten minutes. Into your office comes a patient whom you just finished examining. She settles down in a chair and starts asking questions. You groan inwardly but are I careful to answer her questions. The conversation is mercifully short and you're on your I way in a few moments. How did you come across to the patient?

That patient may well have gotten a completely different impression of you from the one you intended. Your intention was to be efficient in the conversation, spending enough time to answer her questions and make her feel you care about her problem, but she may have perceived you as short and rude. Why? Because of your own nonverbal leakage.

As you spoke you may have been guilty of these errors:

Talking while writing, arranging papers, or doing something else.

Talking while pushing back your chair, standing up, or just sitting back and shifting your legs.

Glancing at the clock, your watch, the traffic outside the window, or other indicators of how much time it would take you to get where you're going next.

Nonverbal leakage is a term referring to unconscious signals that we'd rather be doing something else. Looking at your watch, shifting from leg to leg while you are standing, and looking around at others while the patient is talking are all signals that can convey a negative image. If you intend to withhold your suspicion of a diagnosis pending further tests, be careful not to leak nonverbal cues that would unnecessarily alarm your patient or even generate distrust.

Special Challenges in Patient Communication

Defusing Angry Patient Situations

When you have an angry patient the most important thing you can do is listen. The most harmful thing you can do is counter every charge with a statement or rationalization of your own. Here are some tips:

Give the patient time to talk. Let her say whatever she wants. Look her in the eye; give her encouraging cues to keep her talking; and send nonverbal signals that show you're interested in what she's saying.

When the patient is through, wait. There may be something else she wants to say, and by giving her the chance, you're allowing her to thoroughly vent her anger or frustration.

Next, select a point she made and restate it. Even if you got it all the first time, this technique will show that you truly did hear it, and show that you're committed to getting everything she said.

Actively listen. Paraphrase by using your own words to summarize what the patient said. Use paracommunication that communicates warmth and sympathy.

Remain neutral. As difficult as it may be, don't get defensive or hostile. That will only fuel the fire.

When she's through venting, and you've reflected back your understanding of the problem, then attempt to explain or discuss. Again, use mirroring to reestablish rapport.

Often, this is all that's needed. Perhaps the patient just wanted to get your attention and bring the problem out in the open. Sometimes, though, she will want some action. In that case, go to the next step.

Don't promise anything. Simply say you'll look into it and get back to her within 24 to 36 hours. Then, do it.

Communicating Bad News

Although the practice of medicine can produce the greatest positive experiences possible, it can also produce the greatest challenges. One such challenge is the "right" way to inform a family that their loved one has suffered an unexpected injury or has died, especially if the outcome is unexpected. Even communicating bad news regarding a diagnosis or prognosis is a challenge, the more so if the physician is anxious about what to say and how to say it.

Is there a "right" way to communicate bad news? No one technique will work for everyone. However, there are some techniques that, experts agree, usually work well.

Don't avoid the family. If the patient died unexpectedly, or if something has gone wrong and there is a poor or unexpected outcome the family must be told as soon as possible. They will find out soon enough otherwise, and will hold the physician responsible for shirking his or her duty by not telling them directly.

Take the family to a private room if at all possible. Having a conversation of this nature in a crowded OR or ICU waiting room violates confidentiality as well as sensitivity. If you must communicate in front of others, gather the family around you and speak in a tone low enough so you can't be overheard, but loud enough so that the family can hear without straining.

Don't dance around the subject. They are anxious and probably have a sense of what's coming.

Be compassionate but forthright. A void euphemisms unless you are absolutely certain they won't be misinterpreted. A surgeon, for example, told a woman that her husband "was no longer with us". She thought he meant the patient had been transferred to another facility.

Take your time. Sit down if at all possible. The family will have questions, but it may take them a few minutes to formulate them. Resist the temptation to tell them the bad news, sit for a few minutes, and then leave. If you absolutely must leave, tell them why and when you'll be back to talk more. Find out where they can be contacted at a specific time. Then, make sure you do contact them.

Don't point fingers or admit fault. If the family wants to know what happened, tell them the truth in lay terms. Keep in mind the new standards of the Joint Commission on Accreditation of Healthcare Organizations (JCAHO) that require health care providers to clearly communicate with patients and family members about the consequences of treatment, including unexpected outcomes.[44] It's a good idea to seek guidance from your hospital's risk manager or from your malpractice insurer's risk management department.

---

44 *Comprehensive Accredirorion Manual for Hospira ls, Joim Commission on Accredirarion of Healrhcare Organizarions,* Oakbrook Terrace, IL, 2001.

Working with Noncompliant Patients

Often when things go wrong, it's because patients do not adhere to your treatment plan. They may discontinue medication without telling you, or may stop doing their exercises, or may take other actions that are not in their best interest. Various researchers have determined that from thirty to sixty percent of patients do not take their medications as 'their physicians have prescribed. The numbers become worse for chronic diseases: between forty to fifty percent of diabetics do not adhere to their treatment regimens, and up to seventy percent of arthritic patients don't follow doctors' medication orders.[45] They have the right to do so, but need to know the consequences so they can change their behavior. Here are some tips on working with noncompliant patients.

Get the patient involved. The "'take these pills until they're gone" approach seldom works. Today's patient prefers to be involved in his own care plan. You can involve the patient by asking questions, showing him how to take medication or do therapy, and asking him how he feels about the regimen. Doing so will show you how much importance the patient places on his personal health care, and will help you identify ways to enhance compliance. You may be surprised at what you'll discover. One physician asked a mother to read medication directions for her child's prescription, and learned that the mother could not read.

Ask the patient what he thinks is wrong. If the patient has one idea and you have another, the disagreement must be addressed in order for the patient to concur with the recommended treatment plan. Resolving these disagreements increases the likelihood that the patient will carry through with your recommendations.[46]

Also, ask the patient to predict potential problems. "What do you think will be the hardest part about doing this?" Confronting problems head on allows both parties to come up with solutions together.

---

45 Dahl R. *How ro get through ro your patients.* Hippocrates 11 (4), 38-40, 43, 44.
46 Ibid.,

Patient education is helpful, as explained above. However, for compliance, concentrate on behavior (actually doing it) and the reasons for doing it, rather than telling them how it works. Most patients don't need to know that their blood pressure medication works by inhibiting the influx of calcium ions during membrane depolarization of cardiac muscle, but do need to know that taking it every day is necessary, not optional.

Educate the 'patient about potential side effects. Tell him what to look out for. and what to do if it occurs. Should he call the doctor right away? Should he wait? Let him know what to do.

Emphasize the consequences of failing to follow instructions. Sometimes patients don't follow instructions just because it's more convenient not to, and they don't believe that anything "really bad" could result.

As simple as it sounds, make sure the patient understands your instructions. A consultant tells of a patient who was told to take Feldene once a day, with food. The patient interpreted that to mean a tablet should be taken with each meal. The patient suffered disastrous consequences and lingered in a coma for fourteen days before she died.[47]

Be realistic in your prescribed regimen. Don't expect patients to take pills at 4:00 a.m. Similarly, be aware of the cost of medication and its effect on patients' budgets.

Try putting your treatment regimen in writing. Many drug manufacturers offer handout material for little or no cost. Go over the instructions with the patient point by point, making notes in the margin or underlining key phrases.

Monitor the patient's adherence in a way that is nonjudgmental and nonthreatening. Instead of asking, "Did you take all those pills like you were supposed to?" ask, "Did you miss any pills since your last visit?" The difference is subtle but important. Patients who feel they are being judged may be less likely to respond honestly if they haven't been compliant.

Remember the power of pos1t1ve reinforcement. When a patient complies with a difficult regimen, tell her she's done a good job.

---

47 Bartlett E. and Rehmar, M. *The difficult patient*. Baltimore, EBA, Associates

It sometimes helps to find out what a patient's personal goals are, and support them in reaching those goals. For example, if a patient enjoys skiing, tell her that what she's doing will get her back on the slopes more quickly.

Consider the benefits of a patient educator, who can make sure that patients understand the medication plan at the start of treatment, and can also help with re-education and reinforcement of the plan when patients haven't been following instructions. A patient educator can also help document attempts to ensure patient compliance, and can do much to prevent patient injury.

What about time constraints? To satisfactorily work through a patient's noncompliance may require a minimum of fifteen to twenty minutes. In today's pressured environment where productivity quotas are becoming common, is it realistic to ask the doctor to devote that much time to a single patient? From a risk management standpoint, the answer must be "yes." Not all patients will require the additional time. Spending it with those who do may very well prevent spending much more time later in rationalizing what went wrong, or preparing a malpractice defense.

Terminating Patient Relationships

Some physicians may find it necessary to terminate their relationship with certain patients. Perhaps the patient is non-compliant and you believe that your continued treatment would increase the chances of a complication or poor outcome. Perhaps the patient is rude or abusive to you or your staff, or maybe you just don't get along.

Any of those reasons, and many others, may be reason to terminate a patient from your practice. If you choose to do so, be sure to follow some specific guidelines to minimize the chance you'll be sued for abandonment.

First, put the notice in writing. The reason may or may not be stated. We suggest that if you are dismissing the patient for a clinical reason, such as non-compliance, you say so clearly in the letter. On the other hand, if you are dismissing the patient for non-clinical reasons, such as a personality conflict, an unpaid bill, or for other non-clinical reasons, don't say it in writing.

A suggested format follows:

Dear Mr. Patient,

As I told you during your office visit this afternoon, you require continuing [therapy/treatment/medication] for treatment of your [condition}. You have missed [four] appointments, and despite our attempts to schedule your treatments at a time convenient for you, you have failed to keep the appointments or to reschedule.

Therefore, I find it necessary to withdraw f om your care effective noon on [date}. If you need emergency care before that time I will treat you; however, in no case will I be available to provide medical care to you after noon on [date}. I will provide copies of your medical record to the physician of your choice, and refer to you to the Medical Center Physician Referral Service or the County Medical Society for assistance in finding another doctor.

Sincerely,
John Smith, MD

The above wording would be appropriate for dismissing a non-compliant patient. The letter that follows would be appropriate for dismissing a patient for other reasons (personality clash, overdue bill, etc.).

Dear Mr. Patient,

This is to notify you that I find it necessary to withdraw as your physician effective noon on [date}. If you need emergency care before that time I will treat you; however, in no case will I be available to provide medical care to you after noon on [date}. I will provide copies of your medical record to the physician of your choice, and refer to you to the Medical Center Physician Referral Service or the County Medical Society for assistance in finding another doctor.

Sincerely,
Sara Jones, MD

How much notice should you give? In states where no law provides the answer, you need to give-the patient a reasonable amount of time to find another doctor. In large cities with many physicians, this may be as little as two weeks. In smaller communities, you should give a little more time, perhaps three to four weeks. This is necessary in order to avoid "abandoning" the patient.

In any case, send the letter by certified mail with return receipt requested, and also by first class mail. The first class letter will be forwarded, in case the patient has moved. The certified letter-will provide documentation that the letter was sent and either claimed or unclaimed. Keep the receipt in the patient's file, along with a copy of the letter.

Medical Team Relationships

The preceding discussion focused on relationships between patients and their caregivers - you and your staff. Just as important as physician-patient relationships is the nature of the relationship between and among physicians, nurses, medical office assistants, hospital employees and others who work with patients. In fact, relationships among these individuals can have a lasting effect on patient satisfaction and the course of the patient's treatment.

What constitutes a "medical team?" One answer may be "those who participate in patient care." However, most people will agree that there are important differences between a group of individuals and a "team." A team is a group of people with a high degree of interdependence geared toward the achievement of a goal or completion of a task.[48] Contrast that definition with what is often apparent in the medical setting: instead of working together, individuals compete with each other to demonstrate superiority or gain recognition from others. Such competition precludes teamwork and can present a liability risk.

Health care traditionally has put the physician in the lead position, with everyone else playing subordinate roles. As medicine has advanced, however, its sheer complexity suggests that no one can know it all or do it all. The growing quantity and quality of registered and certified health care professionals illustrates the scope of the issue: whereas yesterday's health care team may have consisted of a physician, a nurse, and perhaps some technicians, today's team will include medical and surgical subspecialists as well as non-physician experts in fields as wide ranging as diagnostic imaging and CPT coding. Today's medical professionals must be able to operate effectively in a complex team environment, not just as skilled clinicians operating independently.

Consider the real-life scenario summarized m the medical record excerpt contained in Exhibits 1 and 2 on the following pages. Even though the incident occurred over a dozen years ago, the illustration is instructive as an example of what not to do when there is a conflict with another health care professional.

---

48 Parker, G. *Team players and teamwork: the new competitive business strategy.* New York, Jossye-Bass, 1991. p. 17

EXHIBIT 1

DATE OF ADMISSION: 6/5/88

DATE OF DISCHARGE: 6/10/88

PHYSICIAN: Dr. A, MD

29-year-old white female admitted and discharged 6/10/88. Mrs. B is a Para 9, Gravida ![sic], 29 year old Caucasian female who had been cared for by me from early pregnancy with expected date of delivery scheduled as 5/21/88 on dates versus 5/23/88 on ultrasound. She has been seen by me regularly in my office, sometimes 2 or 3 times a week, because of the large size of the baby and her term situation. She is A-, Du-, was given RhoGam by me at 28 weeks. She was seen by me on Tuesday, the week before admission. She was admitted on Sunday, 6/5/88, at 16:45 p.m. by nurse C to Labor and Delivery. She was seen by me a week prior on a Tuesday in Labor and Delivery where a 5 hour oxytocin stress test was performed by me which was absolutely normal with no decelerations and no evidence of any placental insufficiency. She had been charting fetal movements since 36 weeks of pregnancy, and returned these each week to me in the office and these had all been normal. Having been submitted to a 5 hour oxytocin stress test, had not gone into labor and the cervix was unchanged, no decelerations, she was told that an induction of labor would probably be unsuccessful and therefore she would go home and continue her thrice daily fetal movement charts and see me three days later on Friday morning, prior to the weekend.

She returned to see me Friday morning. 6/3/88, in my office and the only abnormal finding was 1/2 lb. weight loss. She, however, informed me she had been very active, had not been eating and trying to do a lot of walking to stimulate the onset of labor. I advised her not to do this, that this would decrease the effective placental circulation, that she should rest and really wait for the onset of labor.

I also warned her on 6/3/88 as she was close to dates to count fetal movements three times a day and if they dropped below 10 an hour to notify me immediately or to come to Labor and Deliver). I also notified her that if there were excess fetal movements, ruptured membranes or early onset of labor to come straight into Labor and Delivery, which she intelligently agreed to do. She was a very cooperative, intelligent patient and had totally observed and followed all instructions which I had given her during the pregnancy. She had had a glucose tolerance

41

test at 28 weeks, which was normal. Apart from this, her pregnancy course was uneventful. She apparently arrived in labor at 16:45 p.m. on 6/5/88. I had informed her that if she would notify me, I would come and assess her situation, even if I was not on duty, as I did with my other patients, and if she was in labor, I would deliver her. When her mother asked for them to call me, she was told by the nurse in charge that I was not on duty and therefore they would not call me. This is a very unusual situation and when I asked the nurse on duty why she did this, she said she did not know but probably did it because she thought I was at home with a sick wife, which in fact was partly true. However I was not notified and the patient was allowed to labor and was seen later that evening by the doctor on duty, who assessed fetal distress and did a cesarean section. The first notification I had of this patient having had the infant was when I arrived in my office at 9 a.m. on 6/6/88 and was told that the patient had delivered with no complications, because we had not been notified of any complications. I arrived to see the patient at mid-day and found the patient in intensive care in the nursery and then I managed to unfold the rest of the story. I notified the administrator of my displeasure at not having been notified of the patient's admission, told him that I could understand no reason why this patient, of all patients, was different than any of my other patients whom I was always notified about, and told him that I would want a full investigation of this situation. The patient, however, did well postoperatively and she was discharged home to see me in one week's time. Her child, however, has been transferred to Medical Center Neonatal Intensive Care Nursery and further follow-up of this case will have to take place in further dictation.

Dr. A, MD

Note: Names and other identifying information have been purposely changed or omitted to protect the privacy of the individuals concerned.

EXHIBIT 2

Discharge Summary

Dr. A. does not have any standing orders about seeing his own pts. Frequently he will state that he promised a patient he would come in for her. However, nurse L. had not heard from Dr. A that weekend and dealt with the dr. on call, Dr. M. Dr. M also had no idea Dr. A wanted to take care of this patient. The patient reportedly asked if Dr. A was on call and readily accepted Dr. M.

After delivery Mrs. B. stated she was extremely happy with her care. She reported this to Dr. M and Dr. E., her anesthesiologist at the time of delivery.

_____,RN

Such situations are not uncommon in health care. By its nature, ours is a life-and-death environment. Stress and conflict are common and how they are handled is critical. One key is to handle such conflicts via a proven "conflict resolution" process or through other appropriate means set up within the hospital or the clinic. *Don't document your aggravations in the medical chart.*

The Role of Teamwork

"Teamwork" has been the subject of hundreds of empirical and descriptive studies over the years. Such pioneers as Douglas MacGregor[49], Kurt Lewin[50], Rensis Likert[51] and Chris Argyris[52] have published models for effective team and group behavior and have observed examples of ineffective teams. Blake and Mouton[53] spresented a model for leadership which studied effective leaders and their interaction with groups. More recently, obstetrician Stephen Prather, MD built upon Blake and Mouton's work with his analysis of group behavior in the medical setting.[54] Prather distinguished six elements of physician leadership: communication, acquiring knowledge, decision making, conflict resolution, initiative, and critique and feedback. The manner in which each element is performed depends on the physician's behavioral tendencies, or styles of behavior. Styles range from autocratic ("Do as I say and you'll get better; otherwise find yourself another doctor") to laissez-faire ("If you don't want to follow my instruction that's okay, I still like you"). All of these models are useful in analyzing components of group behavior and effectiveness.

Dimensions of team behavior include:

Climate. Team climate is the interpersonal atmosphere in which members operate. Climate may be characterized as cold, hostile, warm, inviting, open, receptive, relaxed, or tense.

---

49 MacGregor, OM. *The human side of enterprise.* New York, McGraw-Hill, 1960.
50 Lewin, K. *Field theory in social science.* Njujork, Harper&Row, 1951.
51 Liker!, R. *New pallerns of management.* jujork, McGraw-Hill, 1960.
52 Argyris, C. *Integrating the individual and organization.* Njujork, Wiley, 1964.
53 Blake, R. and Mouton, JS. *The managerial grid.* Hjuston, Gulf Publishing, 1964.
54 Prather, S, Blake, RR, and Mouton, JS. *Medical risk management.* Oradell, J, MEdical Economics Press, 1990.

Discussion is the extent to which members are free to discuss matters of importance. Effective teams encourage discussion among all members and invite more reticent members to participate. Ineffective teams allow one or two members to dominate discussion and discourage further participation through subtle or overt messages.

Mission. Effective teams have a sense of purpose. This mission is understood and accepted by all members and serves as the focus for discussion and actions. Ineffective teams lack clarity about goals and often get caught up in trivia or day-to-day activity without determining how that activity may help the group in its mission.

Respect for others is a hallmark of effective teams. Members feel free to offer suggestions without fear of being "put down." Ineffective teams have members who may have their own personal agendas and frequently put themselves first to accomplish personal, not team, goals.

Disagreement happens in every team; how it's handled distinguishes the effective from the ineffective. In effective teams, disagreement is perceived as healthy and is handled by openly promoting discussion on the topic. In ineffective teams, disagreement is often suppressed out of fear of conflict, or if not suppressed is allowed to produce open warfare, pitting members against each other.

Decision-making. Effective teams reach consensus about decisions and are cognizant of what consensus involves. Ineffective teams allow unilateral decisions to be made by real or perceived leaders, or allow the majority to overrule the minority.

Self-assessment is periodic, voluntary and standard in effective teams, which find it instructive to determine how well they are functioning. Ineffective teams do little constructive self-assessment, but will allow finger-pointing and unproductive discussion about "why things don't get done around here."

In the medical environment, teams can appear in any number of settings. In the office, a team may consist of physician(s), RNs, L VNs, receptionists, billing coordinators, office managers, therapists, technicians, and other staff members. The same members are present in the hospital with the addition of new players: consultants, administrators, engineers, support people and other hospital staff.

Common to all is the patient. Too often the patient is not part of the team. However, it's reasonable to place the patient within the team as a viable member, especially in light of the therapeutic alliance that must exist in order for the patient to get well.[55]

With such an array of individuals it's not unexpected that members will perceive their roles differently. When those differences lead to conflict the team must be able to handle the conflict constructively.

In order to maximize effectiveness, teams must have members multiple viewpoints, multiple abilities, and a variety of outlooks. Therefore, it is imperative that all members understand how to communicate effectively, share ideas, handle disagreement and conflict, and reach consensus.[56]

As the physician, you are the natural leader of the medical team. Responsibility for team development rests with you. It is a critical function:

A smoothly-functioning team is better able to serve the patient, thus enhancing quality in perception as well as quality in fact.

Members of a smoothly-functioning team experience greater job satisfaction.

The smoothly-functioning team is much less likely to create situations which present malpractice risks.

A good team is better able to handle emergencies and other sensitive situations which affect outcomes.

To develop your medical team, certain precursors must exist:

You must understand how people tend to interact with others.

You must be able to facilitate the constructive resolution of conflict. *Conflict will develop.* Its handling will be critical to the team's success. Protocols should be in place for handling dissonance.

Team members must understand their roles as individuals and as team members. They must understand the team's goals and aspirations and how they contribute to its success.

---

55 Gutheil et al. Malpractice prevention through the sharing of uncertainty. N Enlg. J Med 1984.; 311 (1);49/51
56 For information on team development workshops call or write to *Medical Risk Management,* Inc. at (800) 728-2375, 2500 City West Boulevard, Suite 300, Hjuston, Teksas, 77042.

How people interact. The physician is the natural team leader. She or. he is the person in charge who is ultimately responsible and accountable for the actions of other team members. Consequently the physician is the one who must facilitate understanding and teamwork among different members with different team styles.

Conflict resolution. Conflict will occur. If it is suppressed, members will likely perceive a lack of respect for differing points of view, and may become disgruntled at the "suppresser." On the other hand, if conflict is encouraged without a constructive framework for handling it, it is possible that it will get out of hand and lead to open warfare. Therefore, the team leader must understand the value of activities that can facilitate constructive resolution of conflict, and should have experience facilitating conflict resolution in the medical setting.

Understanding team roles. Some organizations pay lip service to the idea of teamwork. When new staff members are hired they are welcomed to "the team." However, *how* particular individuals play a part in making the team work is seldom explained satisfactorily. For a fully functioning team to operate smoothly, individuals must understand their own roles and how they, and their roles, interact with others to achieve team goals.

Unfortunately, none of the above skills are innate nor are they taught in medical school. Medical school encourages competition, not cooperation and too often physicians model their behavior after mentors who may be brusque and overly task-oriented. As a result, they may lack skills that can be used in team development and management.

Patient Relationships: One Final Note

At the beginning of this chapter the point was made that most malpractice suits are rooted in a breakdown of communication or relationships. Do patients turn into plaintiffs just because of communication problems? The answer: sometimes. Patients and family members may become angry enough about the way they're treated to seek out an attorney to intervene. No competent plaintiffs' attorney will file suit alleging poor communication, but he or she may look into the situation for their client. The result? The physician receives a letter from an attorney requesting records, and many times the physician's insurance company may end up paying medical and surgical bills, just to avoid a lawsuit.

Case Study #1

Karen Martin made an appointment with a new physician when she developed cramps and heavy bleeding. After the exam the doctor told Karen she had fibroids, and told his nurse to schedule her for a hysterectomy. Karen, who was 41, asked for an explanation and instead of responding, the doctor gave her a book on hysterectomies. She asked if she was at risk of ovarian cancer, and the doctor responded, "If you're concerned about that we can take your ovaries out too." Karen left the office feeling humiliated and scared.[57]

Which of the following more accurately describes the source of the communication problems here?

The doctor gave her the information she really needed. If Karen had taken the time to read the book and accept the doctor's recommendations, all of her questions would have been answered (see #1 below).

The doctor did not give Karen the information she needed. She was specific with her requests, but he was not responsive to her questions (see #2 below).

Both Karen and the doctor shared blame for communication problems. If she did not get from him what she needed she shouldn't have left as she did. If he did not understand what she really wanted, he should have asked her to clarify her concerns (see #3 below).

Discussion

#1 *You said that Karen was to blame for the communication breakdown and that the doctor gave her what she needed.* We disagree. She was clear with her concerns but the physician did not address them. Instead of answering her questions about fibroids, which would have addressed her question, he gave her a book that addressed treatment. Instead of answering her questions about ovarian cancer, he recommended a quick solution. Efficient? Maybe, but at great risk of alienating his patient and increasing his liability if something were to go wrong.

---

57 *How to find a doctor how really cares.* McCall's, June, 1994., p. 46-48

#2 *You said that the doctor was to blame for the communication breakdown.* We agree. Karen was pointed in the information she requested and the doctor declined to provide it, offering solutions instead. There is a time and place for solutions, but an initial request for information about disease processes is not it. He should have taken time to answer her questions, or referred her to a nurse she could talk to, or at least have given her a book about fibroids, not hysterectomies.

#3 *You said that both were to blame.* This may be the "politically correct "answer, but we believe the blame would rest more with the physician in this scenario.

Other issues:

Could the doctor be accused of manipulating the conversation in order to shorten the appointment or persuade the patient to accede to his plan? Possibly. Given the patient's reaction to the doctor's behavior, she'd quickly contact an attorney if the doctor's proposed treatment went awry.

Another issue is her apparent unwillingness to directly confront the physician. She was direct in her requests but unwilling or unable to point out that what she received wasn't what she wanted. This is a common problem when patients perceive their physicians are rushed or uncaring.

A final issue is the doctor's apparent inability to tell the difference between what she asked for and what he gave her. There are discrete steps to patient education including defining the problem, discussing its origins, discussing various treatment plans, and selecting a preferred plan. Karen wanted information (steps one and two), and the physician went straight to step four. Not only does this approach run afoul of informed consent; it also reinforces the perception that doctors are too busy or rude to listen and respond to their patients.

Case Study #2

Refer back to the obstetrical medical record excerpt. Of the following courses of action, what should the physician have done to address his concern about the nursing staff?

He should have told the administrator of the situation and let the administrator handle it (see# 1 below).

He should have documented the incident in the medical record as he did, taking no further action (see# 2 below).

He should have completed an incident report and placed it in the medical record (see# 3 below).

He should have gone to the nurse supervisor over L&D and demanded that the nurse be fired (see # 4 below).

He should have called a meeting to create a forum at which he and the nurses and the supervisor could discuss the incident and take steps to prevent it from recurring (see# 5 below).

He should have documented the incident in a confidential memo to the Quality Assurance Committee (see# 6 below).

Discussion

1 *You said that the physician should have told the administrator of the situation and let the administrator handle it.* Doing so probably would fix the problem in the short term. However, it would do little to resolve the conflict between the physician and nurse; in fact, the conflict and resentment would probably escalate.

2 *You said the physician should have documented the problem in the medical record as he did, taking no further action.* This is one of the worst things he could have done. The physician's anger comes through in the record, casting a shadow on the nurses' actions. Regardless of who was right or wrong, the record remains the key to the case. By pointing fingers at each other, the nurse and the physician have set up a perfect scenario for a plaintiff's attorney, who needs only to capitalize on the conflict to coax a settlement from all parties.

3 *You said the physician should have completed an incident report and placed it in the medical record.* No.

The medical record should be a complete account *of the clinical care* provided to the patient only. It should contain lab reports, admit notes, progress notes, treatment plans, and discharge summaries to name a few documents, all of which are clinical.

An incident report is not clinical. It calls attention to an event that carries some risk and should be evaluated. The proper place to send an incident report may vary from hospital to hospital but chances are it will be the quality assurance/improvement office, department of risk management, or the administrator over safety and risk management.

There is another reason for keeping such incident reports out of the medical record. The medical record can be reviewed at any time by the patient or a properly authorized representative of the patient. It would not be appropriate for the patient, his attorney, or other representative to read confidential incident reports. When they are submitted through proper channels, the incident reports are protected from discovery. Filing them with the record negates that protection.

4 *You said the physician should have demanded that the nurse be fired.* That may have taken care of his problem with the nurse but it wouldn't have done much for the source of the problem, which is lack of communication and lack of respect for each other as professionals. The physician wants his orders followed. The nurse wants to follow orders but first must know what those orders are.

A preferable course of action would have been for the physician, the nursing supervisor and the staff nurses to sit down together as described in option one, above.

5 *You're right.* The best course of action would have been for the physician, the nursing supervisor and the staff nurses to sit down together and agree on how to handle Dr. A's patients in the future, Not much would be gained by rehashing the previous problems; such discussions would probably lead to accusations and denials. It would be more productive to decide as a group what action should be taken with such patients in the future. This should be accomplished by a group decision making process which includes problem identification, problem etiology, possible solutions to the problem, and solution selection by consensus.

6 *You may be right;* the physician should have documented the incident in a confidential memo to the Quality Assurance Committee, if he wanted the incident reviewed and policies set up organization wide. By going through the QA committee, Dr. A will keep the incident and its investigation confidential, because QA committee proceedings are not discoverable in court. Doing so is a good way to focus attention on hospital-wide solutions to problems.

However, Dr. A should still work with the nursing staff to remedy future problems. Going to the QA committee won't help the interpersonal conflict; only the physician and the nurses can address that.

3. MEDICAL OFFICE RISK FACTORS

The preceding section focused on relationships, certainly a critical component of risk management. This section will examine risk factors in the medical office, where nearly 30 percent of medical liability claims originate. 58 Such risks may be procedural (for example, the protocols your assistants follow in pursuing bad debts). Some are systems-based, like the steps you follow in reviewing lab reports before they are filed.

Appointments and Scheduling

Most patients agree that the two most frustrating aspects of visiting the doctor are long waits and high fees. When patients have to endure long waits, they perceive that you really don't care about them, you're indifferent to their needs, and you don't need them. No one likes feeling that way and, if something goes wrong, the patient may well be predisposed to seek out reasons to get back at the doctor. Long waits contribute to the motive for revenge.

What can happen when the schedule is "off'?

Inappropriate scheduling. Does your staff routinely double-book patients? Do you start scheduling patients more than fifteen minutes before you can possibly see them? If so, the results could be a crowded reception area and long waits, prompting patients to think you're disorganized and inconsiderate of their time. Sometimes the problem is unavoidable, as in cases where you have an emergency off-site. Other times it's a matter of miscommunication, as when the doctor doesn't tell the staff that the schedule is different on a given day.

Remember that processing new patients takes time. The staff should recognize that the doctor needs to spend additional time with new patients to inquire about allergies, v medical and family histories, etc. Also, patients should be encouraged to arrive early to fill out forms. If the appointment is for 1:30, advise them it would be good if they were there about 10 minutes early for paperwork.

Set aside some time aside for emergency patients. Also, allow some flexible time for interruptions.

---

58 TMLT Reporter, Vo. 9, No.2.

It's a good idea for your staff to include the patient's phone number beside his name, so he can be readily contacted if an emergency arises. That way, if it's necessary to contact the patient before the appointment, the number will be readily available.

Inadequate time for the physician to spend with patients. If there are too many patients waiting, there may be a tendency to rush through "routine" aspects of a patient encounter like updating the patient's history, inquiring about new symptoms, or educating patients about self-care. Such omissions may contribute to missed diagnoses and patient noncompliance.

Inadequate maintenance of appointment logs. Keeping accurate records of patient appointments is an important part of risk management, since it's critical that you be able to show when the patient was treated and when the patient did not keep appointments.

Here are some tips for managing the schedule:

It's critical to maintain appointment records. If there is an adverse outcome, one of the first questions asked will be, "Was the patient able to see the doctor in a timely manner?" Your appointment book or software will be a valuable aid in your defense, as long as records are maintained properly. Here are some hints:

Missed or canceled appointments should be followed up as appropriate. Some no-shows are critical: those where a patient may suffer if treatment is delayed, or those where you must monitor medication or treatment. In these cases always phone the patient to try to get her back in. If you can't reach the patient by phone or if the patient refuses to come in, send a certified letter to show that you did make the effort. Some no-shows are less important for follow-up: a new patient who skips the first appointment, for example. It's a good idea to call those patients and, if they were referred by another doctor, to notify him or her as well. Document these contacts in the medical record as well as in the appointment log.

Recognize that missed appointments or canceled appointments are often signs of the patient's dissatisfaction with the physician. In addition, liability has occurred because the patient fails to obtain treatment. In such cases the "fault" may rest with the patient for failing to obtain treatment, but defending the case still costs time and money. Clear documentation of missed and canceled appointments may preempt a claim.

Although some patients may skip appointments due to long waits, others may have different reasons. Look to the individuals themselves: the payer mix, the type of appointment (new patient vs. follow-up), and the relative location of your practice to the patient's residence or workplace. Following up with no-shows is good for patient relations as well as risk management.

Never allow missed or canceled appointments to be erased or overwritten in the log. Don't mark through patient names if the patient doesn't keep an appointment. Instead, simply note beside the name that the patient canceled or did not show. You need to be able to document that the appointment was made and not kept.

Keep the logs well past the statute of limitations. If you treat only adults, keeping the logs for five years should suffice. If you treat children, keep the logs until the patient reaches his or her twentieth birthday. Keeping the logs is in addition to documenting no-shows or cancellations in the medical record. Note: these suggestions are for appointment logs. Medical records should be kept indefinitely.

Patient Interaction

Many experts agree that one of the most important types of physician-patient interaction comes during the initial history. During this appointment you can elicit important medical clues that will enable you to plan treatment for the patient. It also provides an opportunity for the patient to evaluate the doctor as a person, based on the quality of human interaction and compassion displayed.

The history is important in medical risk management as well. Studies by the Physician Insurers Association of America (PIAA) have shown that a major problem in cases where the physician missed a diagnosis of cancer was "a serious deficiency" in doctors taking histories from their patients.[59] For example, in 15 percent of cases of missed lung cancer diagnoses, the doctor did not determine if the patient had ever smoked or worked in environments where he or she might be exposed to toxic agents. In 37 percent of breast cancer cases, a family history was not taken.

---

59 *Don 't get sued: missed cancers.* Am Med News, July 25, 1994., p. 15-16

The importance of a thorough history is taught early in medical school. Why might a physician skimp on it? One reason is time: there's pressure to move patients in and out quickly, and the doctor may think he or she knows the answer to the question, so moves on without asking or exploring certain topics. Another reason is the lack of a standard history form to follow. Many physicians ask the same questions routinely and do it by rote. However, if they're distracted or rushed, they may forget to ask some questions.

One solution: Develop a standard history form appropriate to your specialty. Include on it all the information you need in order to evaluate the patient's health. Have it printed and padded (bound together into 50- or I 00-page pads) at your neighborhood copy shop. When you take the patient's history, use that form and make sure that all topics on the form are covered. File the form in the chart. Each time the patient returns for care check the history and, based on your specialty and foreknowledge of the patient, ask if any aspects of the history have changed.

This is a simple device, but effective. It's much better to have a checklist to prompt your memory. Another benefit: the patient can fill out parts of the form you designate, and you simply verify the information orally.

Another critical aspect of patient interaction is follow-up. Following up with patients has many benefits, some beyond strict risk management. For example, the first benefit is increased patient satisfaction. If you treat a patient today and call tomorrow to see how she's doing, she will very likely be impressed with your interest in her well being. If the patient doesn't appear for a scheduled appointment and you or your staff call to see what happened (and document the contact), your liability will be reduced and your revenue may increase when the patient reschedules.

The Office Environment

"First impressions last."

The appearance of your office and the way your office is managed are very important in determining how a patient perceives you. To maximize the positive effect of the office environment, you and your office manager should periodically inspect the office to analyze the extent to which changes are needed. Office inspections should focus on two priorities: patient safety and patient convenience. Patient safety is, of course, a primary concern. Watch out for such potential problems as sharp table comers, worn carpets, wet or highly polished slick floors, electrical equipment, chemicals, medical equipment, glass doors and similar items that can cause personal injury and possible claims.

Risk Factors

Messy or dirty reception area which creates a negative impression. The effect on perceived quality can be significant.

Overcrowded reception area, giving the impression that you are overbooked or backed up and didn't care enough to warn patients so they could reschedule.

OSHA risks, including medical waste disposal, lack of universal precautions, etc.

Premises issues like missing entrance/exit signs for parking lots or lack of equipment for handling snow and ice.

Possible breach of confidentiality due to lack of privacy for examinations or private conversations,

Quality of reading material. Some popular magazines run features like "Why I Sued My Doctor." Be careful what you offer as reading material.

Quality of television and taped material. If you have network or cable TV in your reception area, beware of commercials for personal injury attorneys.

There are special risks associated with children:

Toys that are unsafe, dirty, broken, or inappropriate for age.

Reading material that is inappropriate for age.

No means of calming rowdy situations, especially if parents do not.

Management of Risk Factors

Take steps to make sure the patient's right to privacy is respected. Examination rooms should be configured so that exam tables are not seen from the hallway, where passersby may inadvertently see the patient.

Do not hold conversations about patients or procedures within earshot of other patients. Business areas should be configured so that private medical or financial conversations are not overheard by others. If it is impossible to have a separate office in which to hold financial or other private conversations, use modular furniture to create a separate area.

Make sure prescription pads and syringes are kept out of sight and are never stored in exam rooms.

Designate someone to periodically check on examining rooms and reception areas to assure patient safety and satisfaction.

Step stools of the proper height and sturdiness can aid the patient in accessing the exam table.

Instead of network or cable TV, consider using patient education tapes. Likely topics: wellness, pregnancy (if appropriate for your specialty), heart conditions, elder issues, nutrition, and exercise. Your patients are captive while waiting for their appointments. Why not give them the opportunity to learn about healthful lifestyles or find out about common ailments or procedures?

If you do have TV in your reception area, have it in one area only, so patients who don't want to watch can read or sit quietly without being disturbed.

Telephone, Fax, and E-mail Communication

Today, we use not only the phone, but also the fax machine and email to send and receive information about patients. All are convenient, but all also have some potential pitfalls to avoid.

One of the biggest problems with the telephone is lack of documentation. Document *all* phone communication with patients. If you take or make a call while you are in the office, it is most convenient to pull the chart and document the call immediately. If you are away from your office, use a pocket notepad to write down the nature of the call and what action you took. Alternatively, use a pocket dictation device and have the tape transcribed when you get back to the office. Allow no exceptions: all staff and the doctor should adhere to the same documentation rules.

Other problems arise when the two parties can't make immediate contact. That's when messages are left, and there is potential for miscommunication. Often messages are lost. Sometimes they're received by the wrong person.

Have you ever called a patient and had your call taken by an answering machine? Leaving messages on answering devices presents a potential for breach of confidentiality. You don't know who will hear your recorded message. Try to deal with the answering machine problem before it arises. Ask the patient how she wants you to handle messages if you need to phone her. Or, on your patient intake form, have a place where the patient tells you how to handle phone messages. If you must leave a message and don't have instructions from the patient on how to proceed, it's best to leave a call back message only: "This message is for Ellen Powers. Please call Susan at Dr. Connor's office at 932-9980."

Another telephone issue is that of callbacks. It's seldom that a patient calls and the matter is handled right away. More frequently, the patient is told that the call will be returned. If that's the case, make sure patients are told when to expect the callback-after 5:00 p.m., for example; or over the lunch hour. Many a patient has become frustrated and angry when told, "The doctor is with a patient and will call you back." Unless told otherwise, the patient will likely think the call will come much more quickly - very likely, in ten minutes or so.

It's also important to make sure that urgent calls are handled quickly. The office should have a triage system to separate routine from urgent calls. The doctor, who has ultimate responsibility for the actions of his staff, should establish criteria. Some offices have manuals; others use simple checklists. Whichever method you use, be sure that staff know which calls to refer immediately to the physician (emergencies, other physicians, and specific callers); which can be handled by the staff (nurses, billing coordinator, etc.); and which should be returned at a later time.

What about autoattendant devices? They're becoming more popular in every setting, including medical; however, they present definite risks. Patients in distress should not have to listen to "You have reached the office of Dr. Smith. Press one to make an appointment; press two to speak with the billing department; press three to talk with Dr. Smith's nurse. If you don't have a touch-tone phone, stay on the line. Someone will be with you momentarily." Callers will become even more frustrated, and it's very likely that a jury will feel the same way.

If you must have an autoattendant device, always make the first option instructions on what to do if the situation is urgent. "If this is an emergency, press 8 for immediate response." Will some callers choose that option even if it's not an emergency? Of course-but it's better to handle those calls on a priority basis than to miss a true emergency because someone couldn't get through.

Email and fax communication should be treated as formal communication. Print copies of email messages to or from patients and colleagues and file in the record as appropriate. The same is true for faxes.

Here are some additional tips on handling email and fax communication:

If you must send patient information by fax, always use a disclaimer on the cover stating that the information is privileged and confidential and that the send should be notified immediately if the fax has reached the wrong individual. Also, it's a good idea to telephone ahead to let the intended recipient know that the fax is on the way. And from a risk management standpoint, it's recommended that the recipient be phoned after the fax is sent, to make sure it was properly received. Granted: not every practitioner will be able to adhere to these steps, but those who can will be practicing good risk management.

Computerized Medical Records

Although the "paperless office" isn't yet a reality, computer-based medical records are becoming more common. Potential benefits are significant and include:

The ability to obtain critical information in a timely manner. If a patient is in an accident in another state, the patient's entire chart could be sent via electronic mail to the receiving emergency facility within seconds.

The ability to find information quickly. Instead of flipping through dozens or hundreds of pages and reports, a doctor could search the patient's record for a particular term (i.e., "chest pain") and obtain a report of all instances where that term appears, including the patient's presenting complaint, phone calls, and test results.

The ability to reduce paperwork. From a risk management standpoint, medical records should be kept forever. However, old records are a hassle to store and keep. If records are computerized, thousands can be kept active on your computer's hard disk. Old paper records can be scanned and digitized, eliminating the need for storing old paper records.

Computerized records present drawbacks as well:

Many physicians are not familiar with computers or the programs they run. Although new machines and software programs are easy to learn to use and user friendly, there is still a learning curve associated with becoming computer savvy.

Expense. The cost of moving to a computerized record system can be substantial. Although the price of good computers is coming down, the expense of setting up a single-office network can approach $5,000. For larger groups or sites with multiple locations, the outlay can be significantly more.

Confidentiality concerns. Stories abound about secret information being stolen and disseminated over the Internet or sent to unauthorized persons. These concerns are real. However, the threat of someone walking off with a paper chart is just as real. And good security measures can be implemented by your computer consultant to minimize the threat.

If you have a computerized record system, you need to take certain steps to make sure you protect its valuable information. Here are some tips.

Back up often, preferably nightly. Computerized records are susceptible to a variety of problems: disk crashes, viruses, and inadvertent erasure. Safeguards can be put in place to protect against these.

To protect confidentiality, keep patient records on a file server or computer that doesn't allow outside access. This means that if you have a system using a modem to access outside information services, perform electronic billing, etc., the patient files should be kept on an unconnected server.

Of course, if your purpose in computerizing is to allow access to patient files from outside your office (to share them among multiple locations, etc.), then you must keep them accessible to outside systems. In that case, make sure your computer consultant sets up a security system to prohibit unauthorized access.

Establish different levels of security, so that only employees with "need to know" can access different parts of the record. Your receptionist, for example, should be able to access patient demographic information, insurance and billing information, and other information relative to patient reception and check out. Your nurse, PA or medical assistant will need access to clinical information. And some very sensitive information (HIV and AIDS status, psychiatric information, substance abuse, etc.) perhaps should be accessible only to the physician.

Staff members should have their own access codes for entry into the system. These codes should be kept current, and should be immediately deactivated when an employee leaves the practice. This includes those who resign as well as those who are dismissed. The best access codes and passwords consist of a combination of letters and numbers in a random sequence. Avoid using passwords that may be easily guessed by unauthorized people (for example, "fifi" where "Fifi" is the person's pet's name). Although such passwords are more easily remembered, a more complex password such as "rEp29tv" would be more effective as a security measure.

Make provisions to limit an individual's ability to print the record unless there is an appropriate need for a hard copy.

The system should be able to detect unauthorized attempts to gain access. It should also shut down the system after several unsuccessful attempts to gain access.

Personnel using the computer should log off whenever they leave a workstation. The workstations should automatically log off if not used after a specified time period.

Screens should be positioned so they cannot be read by non-staff.

Guard against modification or alteration. One of the computer's greatest advantages is its ability to facilitate quick, seamless editing of content. From a legal and risk management standpoint, this poses great risk. The possibility that a physician may alter a chart after an adverse event to inaccurately modify events is real. At the least, establish a policy that any corrections will be noted as such, and correctly dated and timed. A better alternative would be to program your software so that changes are automatically documented and noted. Finally, any alteration should be flagged by date and time so that there is no doubt of its source.

Record retention requirements are the same as for paper records. Plan on keeping them for at least two years past the statute of limitations for your specialty, unless the patient is a minor. In that case, keep the records for at least two years past the age of majority, or in accordance with your state laws. Your professional liability insurer may recommend that you keep them forever.

Electronic signatures are generally allowed and accepted.

Informed Consent

Informed is a process, not a form or an event, although many physicians and other health care professionals treat it as an event. The process model of informed consent involves dialogue and two-way communication resulting in an educational and team-oriented outcome. The event model equates obtaining informed consent with obtaining a signature on a form.

Risk Factors

Equating informed consent with obtaining a signature.

Expecting nurses to handle the informed consent process.

Failure to obtain your own informed consent in the medical office (instead, relying on the hospital to do it for you).

Inattention to consent required by law.

Language barriers that remain unaddressed. communication with the hearing impaired.

Documentation of informed refusal.

Management of Risk Factors

Make informed consent a shared decision. Follow the process model by discussing with the patient the risks and benefits of a proposed treatment or procedure; alternatives to a proposed treatment or procedure; risks and benefits of the alternatives; and risks and benefits of doing nothing.[60]

Don't just tell what to expect; ask the patient to feed back to you his or her understanding of what you said. Ask the patient to describe the procedure or tell you what he thinks will happen, for example.

In discussing medical alternatives, do it in language the patient can understand. If the patient doesn't understand English well, speak to him in his own language or get a translator. Translators are not legally required, but having one present certainly makes it easier to communicate. Even if the patient does understand English, speak to him in jargon-free language. Many times patients are intimidated by their doctors, and if the physician is speaking in clinical terms the patient may be too shy to admit that he or she doesn't understand.

---

60 Lidz CW, Appelbaum PA and Meisel A. *Two models of implementing informed consent.* Archives Int Med, June, 1988.

Address the hearing impaired. Some jurisdictions mandate that the doctor must pay for a sign expert. Such experts have three different levels of skill and doctors need to know which are appropriate for certain types of medical consultation.

Document informed consent discussions and patients' decisions, including their informed refusal of treatment, in the office record.

Responsibility for the informed consent process rests with the physician and cannot be delegated. However, physicians often do delegate the task of getting forms signed to a nurse or other assistant. This should only be done after the physician has discussed the procedure, alternatives, and risks with the patient. Under no circumstances should a nurse or anyone else solicit the patient's signature until the physician has completed a full discussion with the patient and/or the family.

Remember: If you ask someone else to obtain informed consent for you, you will be held responsible for what that person tells the patient. That person becomes your agent. Few physicians should be entirely comfortable with that notion.

If a patient refuses to submit to treatment, document that as informed refusal. Forms are available to facilitate this documentation and the patient should sign and date the form.

Finally, include a discussion of your fee structure and billing practices. This isn't technically "informed consent," but it is a subject that should be discussed up front and documented.

Your Office Staff

Your staff probably spends more time with patients than you do. There are hundreds of opportunities for your office staff to interact with your patient. Each of those opportunities is a chance for your staff to enhance your image and your relationship or to sabotage the good you've accomplished. From a quality standpoint, your assistants can create or undo the perception of quality and can also affect quality in fact.

Risk Factors

A busy phone that makes it difficult for patients to get through.

The perception that your assistants are rude or uncaring.

Inadequately trained assistants.

Assistants who knowingly or innocently misrepresent their credentials or your own.

Management of Risk Factors

Educate your assistants to the importance of good patient relations. Make sure your assistants are up-to-date in their technical and clinical skills.

Maintain records of their continuing education. It is important not only for their knowledge, but also to show that you care enough to keep them updated.

Check credentials to make sure your employees are properly and currently licensed. An orthopedic nurse applied for an office position at a busy group practice. She was briefly interviewed by one of the physicians who hired her on the spot. She eventually filled out the usual paperwork but was never asked for evidence of licensure. Six months later one of the physicians was sued. As the plaintiff pursued the claim it was discovered that the nurse had been fired from her previous position due to a problem with narcotics and had subsequently lost her license. In addition to his malpractice claim the physician now had to counter the charges that he employed a drug addict who was practicing nursing without a license.

Don't allow your patients to think that all of your assistants are nurses. It may be easy for you to say "My nurse will take care of that," when you are actually referring to your scheduling clerk; but doing so can lead to trouble. If for some reason a claim is filed, the patient will allege that you are misrepresenting the credentials of your staff. Refer to your assistants by name or by function and alert them to the need to tactfully correct patients who inadvertently call them "nurse."

Information Flow

Communication problems exist in every organization, and in busy medical practices where crises are routine, they often proliferate.

Risk Factors

Not knowing if lab reports are missing.

Filing reports and x-rays without physician review.

Absence of a protocol for handling the flow of clinical information.

Lack of a forum for airing staff members' concerns or questions.

Management of Risk Factors

The physician should review every lab report and x-ray before it is filed. Office protocols should prohibit the filing of any report unless it has been initialed by the physician. That way, the filing clerk will know not to file reports which have"t yet been reviewed.

Many physicians balk at this tip. "There's no way I can initial every lab or x-ray report that comes to the office." Perhaps, but from a risk management standpoint, it's better to take the extra time now to make sure that nothing slips through the cracks than have to take months, later, to defend your missed diagnosis - the one you missed because the lab report was filed before you saw it.

Devise a "tickler system" for following up on lab tests and x-rays. In the tickler, note the deadline by which you should have received the test results or consultation notes. If the deadline passes with no reports, have a system for following up.

Develop and use a system for notifying patients of all normal lab results. Document such notification in the patient's record.

Don't consider it sufficient to send a copy of the lab results to the patient, unless you are absolutely sure that she or he will understand its implications and what to do. An Illinois physician examined a patient whose blood cholesterol test measured at the 324 level. Instead of discussing the results with the patient, the doctor simply mailed him a copy of the report. The patient reasoned that if it had been significant the doctor would have called him. The patient later suffered a coronary occlusion which forced him to take a different job at a lower level of pay. He sued for malpractice. At trial, expert witnesses testified that the patient's high blood cholesterol was a proximate cause of the occlusion and that the doctor's failure to discuss these findings was a deviation from the standard of care. The case was settled for $225,000.[61]

In the same vein, follow a system for notifying patients of all abnormal lab results. Document such notification in the patient's record. Any abnormal lab results or observations should be communicated to the patient only through the physician.

---

61 *A costly lesson in lab-test follow-up.* Med Econ, April 25, 1994, p .. 12

If a particular lab test is ordered, specify that only that test should be performed. It's common today for laboratories to perform a battery of tests on a single specimen and provide the physician with complete results, even though only one or two tests was actually ordered. In such cases, the physician often looks only at the results for the test ordered and ignores the rest. However, if one of the other tests shows abnormal results and the physician doesn't notice or doesn't communicate those results to the patient, he or she can be held liable for failing to notify the patient of a potential problem.

Utilize an internal system for following up with patients who cancel appointments without rescheduling, or who fail to show up for appointments. Be able to demonstrate that an effort was made to get them to come in for their appointments. Document in the patient's chart that the patient didn't keep a scheduled appointment.

For patients who are given medication or appliances, be able to identify and reach them if the need to replace their appliance or medication should arise. Keep the address records current.

Even small practices can benefit from periodic staff meetings. Call everyone together for an hour per month to discuss current events and find out what needs to be changed and how. Such meetings can go far toward building a medical team.

Confidentiality

Remember that communication between the patient and physician is confidential. By extension, communication between the patient and all members of the health care team is confidential. This confidentiality, or privilege, is legally acknowledged in the states. Records of conversations or events pertaining to the patient's care are also privileged, meaning they may not be shared with anyone without the express consent of the patient. There are certain rare exceptions to this as noted in below.

Risk Factors

Disclosure of confidential information without patient's permission.

Release of medical records without express written consent of patient or authorized representative.

Unintentional disclosure of confidential information m casual conversation or electronic communication.

Management of Risk Factors

As a practical matter, no one in the medical office should disclose any information about any patient to anyone outside the office, without the patient's written consent. A patient or a person legally acting on the patient's behalf may authorize the release of confidential information, but must do so in writing, and must specify the information to be covered by the release, the reasons and purpose for the release, and the person to whom the information may be released.

There are certain exceptions to this privilege. It does not apply in a malpractice proceeding brought by the patient against the doctor, in a license revocation hearing, if the patient waives the confidentiality privilege, if the purpose is to substantiate or collect on a claim for medical services, or in any proceeding regarding abuse or neglect of a person in an institution.

Doctors overhear so much that it's easy to tune out most of it. 62 However, patients may strain to tune in on what should be confidential conversations. This includes conversations between staff, your assistant who may be calling in a prescription for another patient, or conversations between you and the patient in the next exam room all which should be private.

The solution is simple: watch your voice volume; pay attention to who else is around and whether they're in earshot; and do a "confidentiality audit" of your office. This involves testing your office and exam rooms to see how easy it is for others to overhear conversations. If you need to install some manner of soundproofing do so; the expense is minimal compared to the cost of placating angry patients and defending lawsuits for breach of confidentiality.

If you receive a call from a person professing to be the patient's spouse, child, parent or significant other, be wary of disclosing confidential information. Even if the relationship is legitimate, the patient still has the right to expect you to respect his or her confidentiality. Even if you think the patient wouldn't mind, you would do well to verify his or her consent before telling the spouse or other person anything about the patient's condition.

---

62 O'Donnell WE. Who's listening? Everybody within earshot.Med Econ, May 9, 1994, pp. 59-65.

If you call a patient and must leave a message on an answering machine or voice mail device, be discreet and don't leave any confidential information on such devices. Remember you cannot control who may retrieve the message.

If you fax patient information to hospitals, insurers or others, remember the same rules apply for disclosure of confidential information. In addition, you must take all reasonable steps to assure that your faxed transmission will be received only by the individual for whom it was intended. Failure to do so may be interpreted as breach of confidentiality.

Remember that even the simple fact that the patient came to the office is confidential. A community physician nearly was sued by a patient angry over the fact that the doctor's receptionist went home one evening and mentioned to her husband that she had seen the patient that day. The nature of the conversation disclosed that the patient had been visiting the doctor; and the patient was angry that such information was being spread without her permission.

It's a good idea to have employees sign confidentiality agreements when they are first hired, and annually thereafter. The annual renewal of the agreement underscores the importance of maintaining patient confidentiality, which will become even more important in the near future.

Office Procedures

Most modern medical offices have office procedure manuals and personnel management guidelines. Such manuals help reinforce staff members' understanding of their office roles, including their risk management responsibilities.

Risk Factors

Not having written policies and procedures or job descriptions. The presence of such documents can bolster your defense if you must explain in court how your assistants are trained or how they are informed of their duties and responsibilities. They are also useful orientation tools.

Inadequate documentation of continuing education.

Lax supervision, due to busyness or complacency.

Management of Risk Factors

Design a written office procedure manual or protocol and keep it readily available for staff members to review.

Develop written job descriptions for each pos1t10n. Detailed job descriptions are not necessary. A simple one-page document per position is fine, as long as it covers the essentials: job function; important tasks or processes; and requirements for completing the job.

Monitor staff to make sure they're not performing services beyond their training or abilities. Only a physician can practice medicine; and it's important to make sure that no other staff members (nurses, managers, etc.) are authorizing prescriptions, diagnosing, etc.

Make sure all staffers know the physician's credentials. There have been cases where a well-meaning staff member told a prospective patient that the surgeon was board certified in a specialty, when in fact he was not. When the patient's results were unsatisfactory, the patient brought suit against the physician, alleging misrepresentation of his credentials.

Billing and Collections

The manner in which your office handles billing and collections is critical, both for your fiscal strength and the quality of your relationships with patients.

Risk Factors

Denying treatment to a patient who is in dire need, because that patient has an unpaid bill.

Surprising the patient with unexpected expenses.

Breaching confidentiality if financial matters are overheard or shared with others.

Alienating the patient with overly-aggressive collection techniques.

Management of Risk Factors

Before their first appointment, let patients know what your billing practices are. Your appointment assistant can do this when she books appointments, by letting the patient know if payment is expected at time of visit, if insurance is accepted, etc.

Discuss fees up front, preferably at the first visit. Most doctors don't discuss fees with patients, but patients want them to.[63]

If you aren't comfortable talking money with the patient, assign one of your assistants to handle the task. Make absolutely sure the assistant's communication skills are top-notch. This is a sensitive area and it is important that the patient does not perceive you as money-hungry.

If the patient balks at paying a bill, discuss it together. Work out an agreeable payment arrangement if possible. If there is an adverse outcome, it is suggested that you don't bill the patient for care related to treating the consequences of the adverse outcome.

If you choose to use a collection agency, give the patient every opportunity beforehand to pay. If you say you will turn the account over to an agency, do it; otherwise you may be accused of harassment.[64]

Monitor collection agency activities. Only those cases for which the doctor has given written permission should result in suit and then, only after the statute of limitations has run.

Medical and Laboratory Equipment

Physicians are frequently named as co-defendants, along with equipment and drug manufacturers, in liability actions arising out of patient injuries involving medical products and devices. In such cases, the manufacturer may attempt to show that the physician or staff were at fault' because they purchased the wrong type of equipment, used the product incorrectly, failed to inspect the equipment for obvious defects, failed to educate the user properly, or failed to maintain the equipment properly.

Risk Factors

Selection of inappropriate equipment for the job.

Inadequate documentation of equipment maintenance.

Inadequately trained staff.

Inappropriate actions taken when equipment malfunctions.

---

63 *Doctors don't discuss feed but should.* Houstin Chronicle, May 30, 1992, p. 10a.
64 Practice management. Med Econ, June 19, 1989, p.43

Management of Risk Factors

Make sure you select the right machine for the job. It is helpful to keep the literature on various options you considered so that you can document your thought processes in choosing as you did.

Train your assistants to use the equipment and interpret its output properly. Document such training and make sure your staffs skills are updated periodically.

Be aware of possible problems or malfunctions attendant to the particular machine. Make sure the operator knows what to expect and how to react.

Utilize an office safety policy on product hazards. Everyone should know what to do in case of electrical fires or equipment malfunctions.

Make sure equipment is used only for the purpose for which it was intended. Doing otherwise will void your warranty as well as increase your liability.

Make sure equipment is calibrated according to manufacturer's specifications and is maintained as required by the manufacturer. Otherwise the manufacturer may be able to assert that the problem was your fault.

If you perform ambulatory surgery in your office, consider complying with all regulatory standards that apply to ambulatory health care centers. You may also wish your facility to become accredited by one of the organizations that certify ambulatory surgery centers, such as AAAHC (American Association for Ambulatory Health Care) or JCAHO (Joint Commission on Accreditation of Healthcare Organizations). Doing so demonstrates your intention to provide highest quality care and can diffuse questions of liability should any arise.

Prescriptions and Drugs

Medication errors and prescribing problems account for a large percentage of medical liability claims. One study revealed that the average payment for a claim based on prescription errors was $120,722. Many of these claims involved serious injuries: quadriplegia; brain damage; even death. Tragically, most were based on simple error: reaching for the wrong bottle; putting a decimal point in the wrong place on a prescription; or overlooking an allergy.[65]

---

65 Crane M. The medication errors that get doctors sued. Med Econ, November 22, 1993, pp. 36-42

Antibiotics are involved in most prescription misadventures. Other drug classes, in order, are glucocorticoids, narcotic and non-narcotic analgesics and narcotic antagonists, NSAIDS and aspirin, and finally topicals, dermatologicals and ophthalmologicals.[66]

Risk Factors

Giving expired drugs or samples to patients.

Lax policies regarding controlled substances.

Informal policies regarding prescription renewals.

Prescribing incorrect dosages.

Not checking for possible interactions with other drugs patient may be taking.

Not asking if the patient may be pregnant or is nursing.

Not checking for allergies.

Management of Risk Factors

Keep literature on all drugs up to date and available in the office.

If you're uncertain about dosage, look it up. For example, you may be accustomed to prescribing morphine or meperidine, but find that the patient can't take those because of allergies or some kind of reaction. Therefore you order another parenteral narcotic. That's fine, but don't guess about the dosage or think it's equivalent. It's not, and the patient could suffer cardiac arrest, respiratory suppression, or hypoxia.[67]

Follow a system for ordering, storing, securing, and dispensing controlled substances in the office.

Take periodic inventory of all drugs. You should be able to tell quickly what your supplies are of each drug and to whom you've dispensed drugs within a given time frame. It's a good idea to maintain a log to record drugs dispensed.

Develop a policy for prescribing drugs and dispensing drugs in the office.

---

66 Ibid.,
67 Ibid.,

Always check current medications before prescribing. It's possible the patient may be taking a variety of drugs from other sources, so don't assume you know what he or she's taking until you've gotten an exhaustive list. Even better, have the patient bring in all of the drugs he or she is taking, including vitamins, aspirin, herbal remedies and other OTC medications. That way you can evaluate for yourself any potential interactions.

Pay attention to allergies. An allergy may be noted inside the chart on the history, but may be overlooked if not flagged or noted on the cover.

Make sure the patient or family member understands what side effects to look for. For example, the long-term use of steroids can result in aseptic necrosis of hips. The drug may be the correct choice, but if the patient doesn't know that the hip problem is a side effect, he or she may not know to report it.

Make sure prescriptions are legible. A decimal point can make a tenfold difference in dosage, resulting in harm to your patient. Never put a zero after a decimal point if your intent is to prescribe a whole unit of medication ("1.0") - if the decimal is hard to see the dosage could be multiplied by ten. Of course, if you are prescribing a partial unit ("0.05mg") you must place a zero after the decimal.

Utilize a security system for controlled drugs. Also, have a system for disposing of expired sample drugs.

Case Study #1

A 28-year-old woman, sixteen weeks pregnant with her first child, came to her obstetrician's office as she was having a spontaneous abortion. The receptionist informed the patient of an overdue bill of $40 and said she would not be seen until she had paid the bill. The patient pleaded that she was in intense pain, in the process of losing her baby, and had no money. An argument ensued in front of the patients in the reception area. The obstetrician heard the commotion, came to the front office and agreed to treat the patient. The patient, acutely embarrassed by the public scene, excused herself to the ladies' room and left, unnoticed, through a side door and went home where she aborted the fetus. She called one of her neighbors for help, and she and the fetus were transported to the hospital by ambulance. She saw her obstetrician at the hospital, where he told her that the miscarriage was unimportant since "it was not a real baby, it was only a lump of tissue." A malpractice claim was filed against the physician.[68]

Which of the following seem to be true statements about this real-life case? Select all that seem true to you.

There was no negligence on the part of the physician (see #1 below)

The receptionist was only following instructions and was not at fault (see #2 below).

The patient should not have been allowed to leave the physician's office (see #3 below).

The physician's words regarding a "lump of tissue" were a precipitating factor in the claim and subsequent settlement (see #4 below).

The physician was accountable for the circumstances leading to the claim (see #5 below).

Discussion

1. You said there was no negligence on the part of the physician, which may be true or false, depending on who is arguing the case.

Technically speaking, it may be argued that the physician was clinically correct in his management of the patient. As soon as he was aware that she was in his office he agreed to treat her without further delay. There was nothing he could have done to keep her from aborting; the abortion was already in progress and could not be stopped. Therefore, strictly speaking, he provided service within the standard of care.

However, it may also be argued that the "standard of care" extends beyond clinical management to interpersonal treatment of the patient. Under that argument the physician, as the individual ultimately responsible for the behavior of those he employs, may be negligent in failing to instruct his staff to accommodate patients in distress by disregarding their financial obligations.

This case did not go to trial, but was settled for $1,000,000. Therefore, the issue of negligence was not decided.

You said the receptionist was only following instructions and was not at fault. Technically speaking you are most likely right.

---

68 Berglund S. *To see ourselves as other see us.* The Pulse, American Physicians Exchange, May, 1992.

The receptionist acts as the agent of the physician, and as such represents him and his policies to the public. Therefore her actions were dictated by her employer; she was not acting independently.

In court, however, it would probably be argued that she "should have displayed compassion," as should be expected of an employee of a caring physician. Therefore, it may be argued that she should have disregarded the office policy regarding payment and allowed the patient to be treated without delay.

Since this case was settled, the receptionist's legal culpability wasn't decided. You be the judge.

You said the patient shouldn't have been allowed to leave the physician's office. We agree.

The patient was under emotional strain and profoundly embarrassed as a result of her progressing miscarriage and the episode with the receptionist. The physician and his staff should have taken immediate steps to monitor the patient closely. His failure to do so would probably constitute negligence, if this case were to be litigated in court.

You said the physician's comment was a precipitating factor in the claim and subsequent litigation. That is true. In fact, it is the primary reason the case was settled. The physician's statement that the baby was "not a real baby, only a lump of tissue" may have been clinically correct. However, that statement completely disregarded the patient's emotional state. She had just lost her baby, and to her, the "baby" was real. To hear it discussed in such callous terms indicated to her that the physician did not care at all about her, the baby, or her situation. Compounded with the incident in the medical office regarding the unpaid bill, the doctor's words were inflammatory and a compelling reason she decided to file a claim.

You said that the physician was accountable for the circumstances leading to the claim. We agree.

The physician was certainly accountable for his own behavior (allowing the patient to leave the office and the statements he subsequently made regarding the miscarriage). As the employer and supervisor of the receptionist he was also accountable for her behavior. He developed, or at least approved, the office policies regarding payment and tacitly or overtly approved of the receptionist's behavior in handling overdue payments.

4. HOSPITAL RISK FACTORS

In November 1999, the Institute of Medicine published its report on medical errors in hospitals, "To Err is Human." According to that report, between 44,000 and 98,000 people die in hospitals each year as the result of medical errors that could have been prevented.[69]

Although the methodology used to arrive at those figures has been called statistically flawed, the reality is that medical errors occur top frequently. Therefore it is no surprise that the majority of events leading to malpractice claims take place in the hospital.[70] Of locations within the hospital, the operating room is the leading site mentioned where incidents occur. The emergency department is also mentioned in a number of suits.

Except for the operating room and ER, there is no one location where claims seem to originate more than others. There are, however, many factors that contribute to allegations of malpractice. Such factors as medication errors and equipment failure play a significant part in malpractice claims. Also of note is the role of communication and information transfer among and between physicians, patients, nurses and ancillary or support staff. Each of these factors will be considered in turn.

Areas of Potential Liability in the Hospital

In general, the following circumstances and events create liability in the hospital setting:

Delays in diagnosis and treatment that exacerbate illness. Such delays may be caused by poor access to care, breakdowns in communication among multiple caregivers including physicians, failure to perform diagnostic tests, failure to refer to specialists, and delay in review and follow-up of pathology, radiology and laboratory results.

Treatment complications, which may be caused by poor assessment or inadequate history.

Adverse reactions to medication, caused by failure to monitor drug levels, liver functions, and renal functions.

---

69 *To Err is Human: Building a Safer Health System.* The Institute of Medicine,November, 1999.
70Professional liability statistics for physicians practicing in Texas. Texas State Board of Medical Examiners, 2002.

Failure to obtain a complete history including information on allergies and medications.

Inadequate informed consent, possibly due to sudden shift from outpatient to inpatient status, the physician relying on the nurse to obtain informed consent, or the physician not adequately explaining procedures.

Inadequate telephone communication, resulting from poor triage and/or lack of telephone protocols, poor communication among physicians, poor communication between managed care plans and the hospital staff, and poor documentation of telephone encounters.

Specific areas of hospital liability are discussed briefly below.

Anesthesiology

Common causes of suits against anesthesiologists include the following:[71]

Injuries involving the placement of the patient. Occasionally a plaintiff will claim injury due to positioning during surgery. Since it is often difficult to prove when the injury was received and who was responsible for moving or repositioning the patient, these claims are often decided in favor of the defendant physician. Complications involving endotracheal tube insertion. Tube misplacement problems are not rare, and the standard of care dictates that the anesthesiologist or assistant must verify proper insertion before notifying the surgeon that the procedure can commence. Failure to detect a misplaced tube immediately will most likely be considered negligence.[72]

Injury to teeth and vocal cords. Although these are unfortunate injuries, they are an inherent risk in anesthesia. The standard of care requires that the largest possible tube be use first, then work down until the proper size tube is found.[73] Additionally, courts have found that patients' teeth could be unusually susceptible to loosening, and that the benefits of anesthesia outweigh the extra force used in its administration.[74]

71 Harney DM. *Medical malpractice.* The Michie Company, 1993., p. 10.
72 *Aubert v.* Hospital "Charity", 363 Co.2nd 1223 (La. App. 1978.)
73 *Bell v. Umsrand,* 401 S.W.2nd 306 (Tex. Civ App. 1966),.
74 *Lemoine v.* Opste bolnice "Bunkie", 326 So.2nd 618 (La. App. 1976.)

Adverse reaction to anesthetic drugs. Virtually all anesthetic agents can produce adverse reactions under some circumstances. Such a reaction does not necessarily constitute malpractice. However, if informed consent is not obtained and verified, the anesthesiologist could be at risk for failing to inform the patient of the possible adverse reaction.[75]

Unexplained cardiac arrest or hypoxia. Neither of these is necessarily an indication of negligence, but can produce troublesome cases for the anesthesiologist if the physician is unable to show that he or she made a thorough pre-operative examination, or if it is shown that the anesthesiologist failed to properly monitor the patient during and after the operation.[76]

Administration of inappropriate amounts of anesthesia. Both too much and too little anesthetic create liability problems. Too much can result in permanent injury or death; too little, and the patient may struggle during surgery and suffer injuries as a result.[77]

Risk Management

Anesthesia is an inherently risky procedure, recognized as such in case law.[78] Plaintiffs' attorneys will zero in on issues of informed consent and negligence.

Make sure that you conduct the process of informed consent in an exemplary manner. Ideally, you should talk to the patient the night before surgery. With same-day admissions that's not always possible. In that case, make an effort to talk to the patient a few days before surgery. Avoid holding "informed consent" talks after the patient has been premedicated. The patient will seldom remember those conversations and the timing makes it easy for the patient to later charge that he or she would never have consented had he or she not been drugged.

Document your actions during and after surgery. This is especially important to show that you were present when you should have been monitoring the patient.

---

75 *Williams v. Menehan,* 191 Kan. 6 379 P.2nd 292 (1963.)
76 *Slayton v. Bruner,* 276 Ark. 143,633 S.W.2nd 29 (1982.)
77 Cezeaux v. Libby, 539 S.W.2nd 187 (Tex. Civ. App. 1976.)
78 *Harney, supra.*

If you suspect a problem with an anesthetic, pull it off the shelves. If possible, send it to an independent laboratory for analysis. Harney tells of a case in which the anesthesiologist sent two vials of anesthesia back to the manufacturer for analysis, but both were "lost." The case settled for a significant sum. Had it gone to trial, the anesthesiologist would have been in a precarious position, since his evidence had disappeared.[79]

General Surgery and OR

The operating room is where 30 to 40 percent of liability claims originate.[80] Leading allegations are surgical complications and negligence including anesthesia (discussed above). Some specific issues are discussed below:

Wrong site surgery. While it doesn't happen often, surgery performed on the wrong site (left leg instead of right, for example) gains attention due to the egregious nature of the problem and the fact that it is I 00 percent preventable. Several professional organizations, including the American Academy of Orthopedic Surgeons, recommend that surgeons sign or initial the correct site prior to surgery in the presence of the patient.[81] Other experts recommend going another step: instead of initialing the correct site, place a special sticker on the wrong site that clearly indicates the site is not the right one.

Improper management of appendicitis. Many surgeons prefer to go ahead and take out the appendix,[82] while others prefer a more conservative approach with antibiotics.[83] Whatever your choice, document your rationale and why you ruled out other alternatives.

Gallbladder surgery. Common complications, including failure to identify and remove a stone from the common bile duct, or injury to the hepatic or common ducts or blood vessels, do not necessarily constitute malpractice. The best defense is good informed consent: explain to the patient what could happen, and what the consequences might be, documenting the conversation and the patient's verbalized understanding and authorization to proceed.

---

79 Ibid., p.31.
80 TMLT Reporter, Vol. 10, No. 2.
81 *20 Tips to Help Prevent Medical Errors.* Family Practice Management, July/August, 2002
82 *Rogers v.* SAD-a, 216 F.Supp. I, 6 (S.D. Ohio 1963.)
83 *Borne v. Brumfield,* 363 So. 2nd 79, 83 (La. App. 1978.)

Surgery for breast cancer. When general surgeons make their own diagnosis on a referred patient, they may be liable for missing a diagnosis. Therefore, some type of biopsy is necessary. To quote a plaintiff's attorney, "A surgeon who fails to order a biopsy before deciding on a course of treatment for a patient with possible breast cancer invites a malpractice claim."[84] As you might expect, informed consent is doubly important with these patients. The patient should be informed of alternative treatment, and should have the opportunity to ask questions and make an informed decision. Many cases turn on this issue, including cases in which the surgeon operated before receiving pathology reports and cases where the surgery was performed on a patient without cancer but who had an excessive fear of cancer.[85]

Foreign objects left in. These cases fall under the legal doctrine of *res ipsa loquitor* ("the thing speaks for itself). As such, no expert testimony is required, because jurors can understand for themselves that, but for the negligence of the surgeon and the surgical team, the injury would not have occurred. Count sponges and instruments twice. If necessary, take an x-ray to be sure nothing was left in.

Colon surgery. Again, make sure that alternatives are explained and informed consent documented. Document your selection of procedures and indicate why you chose as you did and why you decided to forego other procedures.[86]

Other procedures of note to general surgery include gastric surgery, vein stripping, sigrnoidoscopy and blood transfusions. With these and others, informed consent is imperative.

Radiology

Misinterpretation of films. Missing something on film is not necessarily negligence and the courts allow some margin of error in interpreting x-ray films.[87] Courts are not so accommodating if procedures are in place to double-check interpretations and those procedures aren't followed. Further, if the patient has a previous set of x-rays and the radiologist fails to check those, the radiologist will be held accountable in case of a missed diagnosis.[88]

---

84 Hamey, supra, p. 54
85 *Kinikin v. Heupel,* 305 n.W.2nd 589 (Minn. 1981.)
86 *Purcellv. Zimbelman,* 18 Ariz. App. 75 500 P.2nd 335 (1972.).
87 Francois11. Makrohisky, 67 Wis. 2nd 196,226 .W.2nd 470 (1975.)
88 *Smirhv. Courrer,* 575 S.W.2nd 199 (Mo.App. 1978.)

Ambiguous terminology is another problem. For example, "no definite fracture or dislocation is noted." Is there one or not? Terms like "significant" and "insignificant" also pose problems. If a finding is "significant," the radiologist should be certain that other radiologists would think so, too.[89]

Poor film quality. Sometimes missed diagnoses are the result of poor film quality rather than from human error. Risk management experts recommend that the radiologist should be satisfied that the equipment is in good condition, adjusted for the proper exposure and that the radiologic technologists who run the machines are properly trained.

Failure to report findings. This is one of the leading causes of allegations of failure to diagnose. The radiologist has a duty to report his or her findings to the physician who -ordered the test. If the case is classified as an emergency, the radiologist should call, then follow up with a written report. Failure to report promptly constitutes a breach of duty and juries are notoriously unsympathetic to such communications breakdowns.[90]

Injuries resulting from radiation. In instances where equipment malfunctions or where inappropriate exposures to radiation cause harm, the radiologist may be held liable, along with the manufacturer of the equipment. The same is true of contrast studies where the patient suffers an injury from the contrast media, or where a known complication occurs and the patient was not forewarned.[91]

What if an emergency arises during a procedure? Although the radiologist is a physician, it's generally considered that he or she is an expert in diagnosis, not treatment. Therefore, help should be immediately summoned from a surgeon, internist, or emergency physician. Further, if the patient is taking anticoagulants, the radiologist should make sure a surgeon is readily available in case of emergency or immediate complications.[92]

---

89 *Tams v. Kolz,* 530 a.2nd 1217 (D.C. App. 1987.)
90 *Phillip v. Hospital* "Good Samaritan", 65 Ohio App. 2nd 112, 416 .E.2nd 646 (1979.)
91 *Haven v. Randolph,* 342 F. Supp. 538 (D.D.C. 1972)
92 *Marson v. Naifeh,* 122 Ariz. 360,595 P.2nd 38 (1979)

Pathology and Laboratory

Like radiologists, pathologists have a duty to perform their diagnostic functions within the standard of care. Like radiologists, their duty is to examine and report. Generally there is no patient-physician relationship. However, that lack of relationship doesn't protect a pathologist or laboratory from liability if negligence causes harm to a patient.[93]

An error m interpreting specimens doesn't necessarily constitute negligence, even if the mistake results in unnecessary surgery. However, if the mistake results in permanent injury or death, and if the disease could have been treated earlier had the mistake not been made, then the pathologist will have a challenge in asserting that he or she was not negligent.[94]

A common problem is delay or failure to report results. The standard is to report results immediately when critical limits of specified test results are exceeded. If a pathologist's failure to report results produces a significant delay in diagnosis or treatment, there's a good chance that he or she will be found negligent and guilty of malpractice.[95]

The Emergency Department

Empirical data shows that the ED is named in a relatively low number of claims (from about 8 percent to about 15 percent of claims).[96] However, it's a volatile setting. Stress is high (especially in trauma centers) and patients and family members feel out of control.

Some areas of specific concern in emergency medicine are discussed very briefly below.

---

93 *Latson v. Zeiler,* 250 Ca. App. 2nd 301, 58 Ca. Rpn. 436 (1967).
94 *Lauro v. Travelers Ins. Co.,* 261 So. 2nd 261, 267 (La. App. 1972)
95 *Garrison v. Medical Center of Del.,* 581 A. "nd 288 (Del. 1989)
96 *Professional liability statistics for physicians practicing in Texas.* Texas Stale Board of Medical Examiners, 1992.

In-house emergencies. Because emergency physicians have special expertise in CPR, they frequently assess and treat patients in emergent conditions who are not in the ER at the time. As a result, these physicians are exposed to double liability: from the patient who is treated on the floor or in the special care unit, and from the patient in the ER who is not treated because the emergency physician is elsewhere.[97] To manage this risk, the emergency physician should define his or her responsibility and make sure it's part of the contract with the hospital. It should include a section on handling in-house emergencies. Also, the emergency physician should make sure his or her liability insurance covers assistance given outside the ER.

House staff. Expertise of emergency medicine residents varies. A fully licensed, experienced emergency medicine faculty member, along with the first-year resident, must actively assess every emergency patient. Second year residents can theoretically practice unsupervised; however, since they are expected to exercise the same judgment and skill as fully licensed and practicing physicians, close monitoring should continue.[98]

Consultations. The courts recognize that the emergency physician's role is to stabilize and treat until the appropriate consultant can take over.[99] Therefore, the standard of care requires that the appropriate consultant be called and noted on the chart. However, some hospitals require that the patient's personal physician be called first. From a risk management standpoint, if calling the personal physician first would hinder the process of getting the patient appropriate specialized care and the patient would suffer, such a policy should be not be followed because it puts the patient's needs second.[100] If consultation is obtained over the phone, the emergency physician is at risk because the consultant hasn't personally examined the patient and may give an erroneous opinion.

---

97 O'Riordan, WO. In-house emergencies. Emergency Medicine Risk Management, American college of Emergency Physicians, 1991, pp.253-259.
98 O'Riordan, WO. *House staff.* Emergency Medicine Risk Management, supra, pp. 261-265.
99 *Dalgo v. Landry,* 424 SO.2nd 1159 (La. App. 1982)
100 *O'Riordan,supra.*

On-call lists. Most hospital on-call lists are used by the emergency physician to call in experts. If the on-call physician doesn't respond in a timely manner (usually within thirty minutes), the patient as well as the emergency physician is at risk. If the on-call physician doesn't respond, the emergency physician must be able to take alternative means of securing care for the patient. 0 'Riordan suggests having the medical staff formalize a policy on the subject.[101] If there is conflict between the on-call physician and the emergency physician regarding treatment and the conflict cannot be resolved among the physicians, the patient's family should be informed and given the opportunity to accept one opinion or another, or secure a second or third opinion. Of course, the disagreement should be objectively noted in the chart, along with the patient's or family's response.

Other emergency department risks include admission procedures, telephone orders from private physicians, discharge, disposition and follow-up, patients who leave AMA, triage, and a host of other matters. For an excellent clinical and risk management discussion of these and other emergency medicine medical-legal matters, see Emergency Medicine Risk Management, published by the American College of Emergency Physicians.

Informed Consent

The importance of informed consent cannot be overemphasized. Too many physicians treat it like a formality, often omitting it altogether. Why? There are several reasons:[102]

The perception that patients do not want a lot of information. One orthopedist told us that patients get nervous when they are given too much clinical information about a procedure. Tip: If the patient says, "That's enough; don't tell me any more," write that in the chart.

Ideally, have the patient sign a statement saying he or she doesn't want to hear the risks and benefits.

The perception that patients will ask for information if they want it. That's not necessarily so; many won't ask for fear of looking ignorant or for fear of taking too much of the physician's valuable time. This is especially true when physicians give verbal permission to ask questions but use body language that strongly discourages it.

---

101 Ibid.,
102 Skelly FJ. *The payoff of informed consent.* Am Med ews, August I, 1994.

83

Paternalism-the physician's perception that "doctor knows best." This is dangerous on two counts: first, the patient doesn't get to hear about alternative to what you plan; and second, if you come across as arrogant or condescending a patient may well become irritated or frustrated.

Do not assume that informed consent has been taken care of because a nurse obtained a signature on a form. Only the physician can obtain informed consent. Nurses or support staff can assist with documenting the process by obtaining the patient's signature, but the signature does not necessarily mean that informed consent has been obtained. It only means that the patient has signed a form. Remember: informed consent is a process-a dialog between the patient and the physician. Unless that dialog has taken place and the patient truly understands the risks and alternatives, there is no true "informed" consent.

If "informed consent" is obtained after the patient has been prepped and medicated, you should understand that there is strong evidence to suggest that no real informed consent was obtained, even if the form was signed. Likewise, if the patient changes his or her mind and withdraws consent, you should accede to his or her wishes unless there are extenuating circumstances.

Medication Errors

Medication errors account for about 10 to 15 percent of claims. 103 They present problems not only in the physician's office but also in the hospital.104

Risk Factors

Drug allergies.

Failure to give adequate instructions.

Illegible orders/prescriptions.

Ignoring side effects.

Inadequate monitoring.

---

103 *Drug administration errors in infants: don't blame individuals,fix the system.* Drug and Therapeutic Perspectives 15 (9): 11/13, 2000.
104 Crane M. *Prescribing habits that will land you in court.* Med Econ, Vol. 67, No. 18, September 17, 1990, pp. 54-57

Management of Risk Factors

Listen to the patient. Many times the patient will let you know about allergies, adverse reactions and other medication-related issues, but if you are making notes, reading the chart or "tuning but" you won't hear the patient.

Review the chart and pay attention to noted allergies. Although it sounds simple, too many physicians either ignore or just don't see allergies the patient has already cited. Other times, the physician may not want to change a medication order even when reminded of an allergy, on the grounds that the prescribed drug is the best for the condition. If so, be prepared to prove your case. Document!

Tell the patient what you're giving him and what you expect the drug to do. Also, clarify potential side effects or reactions. This serves two purposes: it protects you and also gives the patient a better idea of what to expect. That way, if there is an adverse reaction, the patient is prepared and knows the appropriate steps to take.

Make your orders legible and understandable. Some drugs sound alike when verbalized: "Zantac" and "Xanax," for example. When writing your orders, don't use a zero after a decimal. If the decimal isn't seen, the dosage may be increased ten times. By the same token, always use a zero before a decimal. The exception: if you're writing an order for a dosage which must be expressed in partial units (i.e., ".05 mg Synthroid").

Taking advantages of technological innovations can reduce prescribing errors. As long as complete information about the patient is in the system, these devices can provide valuable assistance in prescribing medications.[105]

If you treat children, specify pediatric dosages when necessary. Otherwise a child may be given a full adult strength dose of medication.

Also, be aware that there are pharmacokinetic differences in infants compared with adults. Examples include greater absorption of drugs through the skin, slower and more erratic gastric emptying, altered volume of distribution due to different body composition, and reduced clearance as a result of less mature hepatic processes.[106]

---

105 Medication Errors Symposium White Paper. Physician Insurers Association of America, Rockville, MD, 2000.
106 Drug administration errors in infants: don't blame individuals, fix the system. Drug&Tl1erapeutic Perspectives 15(9): 11-13, 2000.

Specify the mode of administration. There was a case in which a physician had given orders that all medications were to be given IV. A nurse took his orders literally and administered Maalox intravenously. The patient died.

Medical Equipment

In today's high-tech world we rely on machines to diagnose, monitor, treat, and perform many sophisticated medical procedures. When the machines malfunction, the results can be devastating.

Risk Factors

Non-compliance with the Safe Medical Devices Act.

"State-of-the-art" equipment.

Lack of procedure for handling malfunctioning equipment.

Untrained or unsupervised hospital staff.

Re-use of single-use medical devices.

Management of Risk Factors

The Safe Medical Devices Act requires that hospitals report to the Food and Drug Administration (FDA) information which "reasonably suggests" that a medical device has caused or contributed to serious injury, serious illness, or death of a patient at that facility. The Act does applies to both physicians' offices and hospitals. However, you should know that if a machine malfunctions in the hospital, you may be involved in an incident which may be reported to the FDA.

Beware of "state-of-the-art" equipment - not because it may be superior or otherwise, but because calling it that may imply that it's the most current available. If you admit a patient to a hospital for a cardiology workup and the hospital promotes itself as a state-of-the-art heart center, it could be argued that the patient had the right to expect that all the equipment would be the newest and best available. If that's not the case, don't tell the patient that he or she will be evaluated by "state-of-the-art" equipment.

If a machine malfunctions, remember that both you and the hospital owe a duty of care to the patient. If there is an obvious defect and you use the machine anyway, you'll probably be held responsible. If the defect is less obvious, liability may rest with the manufacturer and/or the hospital.[107] Therefore, when equipment malfunctions take it out of service and have a written evaluation prepared by an independent biomedical technician. Only then, allow the equipment to be repaired; otherwise you may be depriving yourself of key evidence.

Many hospitals reuse medical devices that are intended for one-time use only. They do so in part to save money and in part to avoid creating waste.[108] The Food and Drug Administration (FDA) has been given the responsibility for regulating this practice. The FDA is addressing the issue by providing guidance for hospitals and reprocessors on such reuse of single-use devices. The guidelines are fluid and subject to change, so it's a good idea to keep abreast of the latest, which are posted on the FDA website.

Case Study #1

The patient was a healthy 36-year-old man who had been referred to a well-qualified otolaryngologist for a tonsillectomy. When the surgeon arrived in the operating room, he noted that the patient's chest was not expanding and retracting even though an endotracheal tube had been inserted. The surgeon placed a stethoscope to the patient's chest and found no signs of ventilation and pulled the tube out. However, he decided to proceed with surgery and the patient was reintubated.

After removal of the first tonsil, the surgeon noted the blood in the area was turning dark and asked the anesthesiologist what could be done to "pink up" the patient. At that point, the anesthesiologist increased the amount of oxygen and the surgeon proceed to remove the second tonsil. The blood again turned dark; oxygen was again increased, and the procedure was completed.

---

107 Dahlquist CD. *The impacl of technological advance on risk management.* Perspectives in Health Care Risk Management, Vol. 11, o. 4, Autumn, 1991, p. 7-10
108 Makers lean on hospitala that reuse disposable devices. AHA News, Vol. 34, o 24, June 22, 1998.

After surgery, the anesthesiologist administered an antinarcotic medication to hasten the patient's wakening then removed the endotracheal tube. The patient was then taken to recovery, where the anesthesiologist checked him periodically. The patient still had not regained consciousness after several hours, so the anesthesiologist ordered "stat" blood gases. The hospital took several hours to complete the studies, which showed the patient was suffering from a profound lack of oxygen in his circulating blood. The patient was reintubated, but it was later determined he had been suffering from oxygen deprivation for a long time, which produced severe permanent brain damage. The family sued the surgeon, the anesthesiologist and the hospital.[109]

Which of the following do you think may be the findings of the jury? Select all that apply.

The surgeon was liable, because he decided to proceed with surgery despite the original esophageal intubation (see #1 below).

The surgeon was not liable, because he did what he could to save the patient (see #2 below).

The anesthesiologist is liable, because he was negligent in intubation, in monitoring and in failing to maintain a proper anesthetic-oxygen mix (see #3 below).

The hospital was liable for delaying the "stat" blood gases (#4 below).

The hospital was liable for the actions of the anesthesiologist (#5 below).

Discussion

You said the surgeon was liable because he decided to proceed with surgery despite the initial misintubation. The specifics of how he was petitioned aren't known, but it is known that the jury exonerated the surgeon completely, saying they considered him a hero for yanking out the endotracheal tube in the first place, therefore saving the patient's life.

You said the surgeon was not liable because he did what he could to save the patient. That's what the jury said. Although they had opportunity to weigh his negligence, their verdict was to exonerate the surgeon of all charges, based on the fact that he was observant enough to notice the lack of apparent oxygenation and do something about it to save the patient's life.

---

109 Harney OM. *Medical malpractice,* The Michie Company, p. 9-11.

You said the anesthesiologist was liable for negligent intubation, failure to monitor and failure to keep the patient adequately oxygenated. The jury agreed. They found that the anesthesiologist did not adhere to the standard of care for monitoring. They also didn't care for his primary defense, that if the patient suffered injury it was due to some idiosyncratic reaction to one of the gases administered during surgery.

You said the hospital was liable for delaying "stat" blood gases. Although we think that should have been considered, the jury was more interested in the hospital's liability for the actions of the anesthesiologist. To our knowledge, the failure to return stat test results was not a factor in the jury's decision.

You said the hospital was liable for the actions of the anesthesiologist. That's what the jury said. It found the anesthesiologist was an actual agent (not an "ostensible" agent) of the hospital because the hospital owned all of the anesthesia equipment, scheduled the anesthesiologist's cases, and controlled his work time.

Case Study #2

A radiologist who interpreted an MRI scan of the patient's cervical spine detected two herniated discs, but didn't detect a visible nasopharyngeal carcinoma. Complaining of a stuffy ear, runny nose and difficulty swallowing, the patient was twice diagnosed with sinusitis by the defendant during a two-month period following the MRI. The decedent's carcinoma was discovered nearly four months after the MRI; he received chemotherapy and radiation therapy, but died 3 and a half years later. The cancer was clearly visible on the MRI.[110]

The defense offered two contentions: that the radiologist was not required to investigate the nasopharynx because the test had been ordered by a neurologist; and second, that catching the cancer earlier would have made no difference to the eventual outcome.

What do you think about the above defense strategy? See below for comments.

---

110 *Pfeffer v. Hendricks,* Ventura County (California), Superior Court, Case No 105645.

Discussion

In court, the defense would argue that the standard of care did not require the defendant to examine the nasopharynx because the MRI had been ordered by a neurologist looking for the cause of the neck, shoulder, and ear pain. This defense would be convincingly argued by both sides, and the jury would have to decide which side's experts were "right." Thus, the standard of care would be determined by the Jury.

Regarding the defense that it would have made no difference to the outcome had the cancer been caught earlier, again, contradicting medical facts and opinions would be offered by both sides. However, since lay people are more familiar with the concept of how cancer spreads, this would be an argument that would more likely benefit the defense.

In this case, a defense verdict was reached, based on the two defenses mentioned above.[111]

Case Study #3

A patient with lower back pain and stiffness in his knees sought the advice of a neurologist, who believed the patient suffered from a progressive spinal myelopathy. A myelogram and CT scan were performed to determine the cause of the condition; and an MRI was performed to rule out arterial venous malformation (A VM). The results were inconclusive and the neurologist decided against angiography.

Eighteen months later the neurologist detected a change in the patient's condition, including decreased urinary function and a weakened foot. A second MRI was ordered but was postponed due to equipment failure and insurance problems. Three months later the patient became paralyzed in his lower body. Exploratory surgery revealed a spinal arterial venous malformation; the patient's paralysis was permanent.

The patient sued and a jury found in favor of the neurologist. On appeal, the patient argued that the neurologist owed him a duty of informed consent, in that the patient should have been told what an angiogram was and how it was used as a diagnostic tool, and how it could have been used to exclude the possibility of AVM.[112]

---

111 *Medical malpractice verdicts, settlements and experts.* Vol.lO, No.7, July, 1994., p. 51-52
112 *McGeshick v. Choicair,* 9 F.3rd 1229 (C.A. 7, Wisc.,November 15, 1993)

Do you think the informed consent argument has merit? Support your reasons.

Discussion

The court said the doctrine of informed consent was meant to apprise patients of risks inherent in a proposed treatment, not to provide a patient with all the knowledge a physician may have regarding a patient's condition and possible treatment. The court concluded that, under the doctrine of informed consent, a patient is not entitled to all the information a physician possesses. The trial court's decision was affirmed.

5. RISKS ASSOCIATED WITH MANAGED CARE

Many physicians say the practice of medicine used to be relatively uncomplicated. A doctor graduated from medical school, completed an internship and residency, then went into private practice by "hanging up a shingle." Occasionally, two or more doctors would form a group practice, but most physicians were in private practice. When a patient was sick, he or she went to the doctor of choice, paying cash (more recently by credit card) or even by barter. If the patient had insurance, most often the physician would bill the insurance carrier then bill the patient for any balance. And, most likely, the patient would pay.

The above scenario can still be found in the United States today, but it's becoming increasingly rare. Contrast it with what happens today if the patient is insured by a health maintenance organization (HMO), or if insurance is provided by a preferred provider organization (PPO) or other form of integrated delivery system (IDS). All are considered to be MCOs (managed care organizations).

When a patient gets sick he or she likely is seen by a primary care physician, one of many in a freestanding clinic. This physician may never have seen this patient before, and must learn about the patient via other doctors' notes or by reading a computerized patient record. The patient is evaluated and very likely treated at the clinic. If the patient requires hospitalization, mechanisms kick into action to pre-certify the patient and authorize a specific number of days in the hospital. If the patient requires additional days, those must be authorized in advance or the hospital and doctor won't be paid for the additional time and care.

How Managed Care Affects Cost

Proponents of managed care assert that quality of care is maintained and costs are controlled. Certainly the trend is affecting how, and how much, care is provided. In Rhode Island, for example, Blue Cross has implemented new "optimal recovery guidelines" that drastically reduce inpatient hospitalization. Elsewhere, the average for hospitalization for an open cholecystecomy or appendectomy is 7-9 days; in Rhode Island, it's one day.[113]

---

113 R.I. *doctors face 'absurd' inpatient limits.* Am Med News, March 21, 1994.

Even as managed care erodes hospitals' inpatient days, it is having the opposite effect on outpatient services. One study revealed that 93 percent of HMO patients receive GI imaging in outpatient departments, versus 43 percent of the patients covered by traditional indemnity insurance. The same holds true for CT scans, cataract surgery, echocardiography, MRis and ultrasound. HMO patients requiring invasive procedures like angiography, arthroscopy, cardiac catheterization, and sinus endoscopy are being more frequently treated on an outpatient than an inpatient basis.[114]

The 1990s were boom years for HMOs, when membership topped the 70 million mark.[115] A backlash against some of the cost-cutting measures used by HMOs has reduced membership in HMOs but increased membership in PPOs and other group health plans. According to the American Association of Health Plans, the trade group that represents HMOs and other types of health insurers, approximately 170 million Americans are currently members of some type of managed care organization.[116]

Opponents of managed care state that quality of care is endangered by incentives to hold costs down, which in tum may make a physician think twice about referring to a higher-priced specialist or providing necessary treatment. Additional concerns focus on patient relationships. Strong patient-physician relationships are key in making patients less likely to sue; yet the managed care environment threatens that relationship by making it difficult for a patient to bond with a single physician. Also interfering with the doctor-patient relationship are MCO management decisions that drop doctors from managed care networks with little or no warning. In such cases patients who have come to trust and like their doctors are forced to give up that relationship in exchange for continued coverage. Doctors and patients alike are up in arms. As a result, legislation has been passed or introduced at both the state and federal levels to protect patients from arbitrary decisions that have potentially serious ramifications. In 2022, the House of Representatives has passed a patients' rights bill that ensure patient access to emergency room care, medical specialists and that women may see their OB/Gyn physicians without a referral.

114 HMO *Outpatients help keep hospitals afloat.* Hospitals and health networks, June 5, 1994, p. 64
115 *The largest HMOs.* Hospitals and Health etworks, June 5, 1998.
116 http://www.aahp.org/template.cfm?section=About_AAHP.

Managed Care Risks

This section focuses on risks associated with managed care. In general, these can be divided into categories:

Relationship-based risks (disruption of the doctor-patient relationship);

Cost-based risks (incentives to not refer or order tests or treatment);

Tort liability risks (where liability is placed if a malpractice claim is filed).

Definitions

For the purpose of this chapter the following definitions will apply:

Health maintenance organization (HMO): a prepaid health care plan that provides basic health services with an emphasis on primary care. HMOs require the use of participating providers who agree to provide specific health care services to HMO members.

There are different types of HMOs. The staff model HMO directly employs salaried physicians and usually owns or leases its own facilities. The IP A/group model HMO provides prepaid care for members through contracts with individual provider groups, or entities having provider employees. The providers (physicians, nurse practitioners, psychologists, etc.) may treat HMO subscribers and may also treat their own private patients.[117] Although the staff model HMO is the original HMO type, we're seeing more hybrid models like the group/IPA model, and increasing numbers of point-of-service models (POS), in which a member may consult a non-participating provider at any time, paying more for the privilege. The POS plans also have traditional limits on coverage, like usual-and-customary ceilings on reimbursement.[118]

Preferred provider organization (PPO): A health plan with provider choice. Under a PPO plan, a member has coverage with both participating providers and non-participating providers. Services through a participating provider costs the member less. The PPO providers provide these services on a discounted, predetermined, fee-for-service basis. Patients pay premiums to the PPO which, in turn, reimburses the providers for their services.[119]

---

117 Chittenden WA. *Malpractice liability and managed health care: history and prognosis.* Torts and Ins Law J, Vol. 26, No. 3, 451-496, spring,
118 *"Pure HMOs:* an idea whose time may be up. Med Econ, April 25, 1994, p.10
119 Ibid.,

Point-of-Service Plan (POS): A type of managed care plan in which members may choose, at the time services are needed, whether to receive those services through the HMO or through a traditional fee-for-service arrangement.

Each type of plan has its advocates. Judging from the race for patients' right legislation, it appears that strict HMO models will probably yield to hybrid models that will blend traditional managed care practices with more lenient patient-oriented ones.

Relationship-Based Risks

As noted above, a major concern of physicians and patients alike is managed care's potential for disrupting the patient-physician relationship. It is axiomatic that patients who like and trust their doctors are more likely to comply with instructions, adhere to medical advice, and get well more quickly.[120] Conversely, patients who perceive their doctors as strangers, who spend little time getting to know them, and who seldom see the same doctor twice are more likely to be critical of the doctor and of the care they received, and are less likely to be compliant with the recommended course of care.

From the physician's point of view the situation is similar. Physicians know that patients value extended contact with their doctors, but managed care emphasizes expediency and rewards volume. The doctor who ignores those facts and persists in spending quality time with patients will build stronger relationships, but will make less money and may jeopardize his continued participation in the network.

Managing Risk Factors

Before joining a plan, talk to your colleagues. Ask them about the plan's willingness to discuss and resolve patient complaints. If your colleagues' patients are dissatisfied with the plan's responsiveness, your patients will probably be dissatisfied too.

Review the plan's member information material. Is it readable? Is it understandable by the average lay person? These are the rules that govern what treatment is covered, and if your patients don't understand it, they may blame you if they find out too late that certain treatments, devices, drugs or referrals are deemed "not necessary."

---

120 *Avoiding managed core's liability risks.* Med Econ, April 25, 1994., p. 68

The plan should also tell your patients about private fee-for-service options that may be available. Sometimes patients can use member physicians for treatment that isn't covered by the plan. This option should be clear in the member education material. Also, if the managed care plan offers a POS option, its terms should be spelled out clearly.

If you choose to contract with the plan, be familiar with all of this material. If you don't choose to discuss the fine points with your patients, have someone on your staff who's an excellent communicator do it on your behalf.

Check out the plan's grievance procedure. Are records of hearings carefully maintained? Can the process answer questions regarding the availability of medical judgment, when necessary? How are grievances resolved? There should be a standard procedure for handling member grievances that deal with questions like this.

Finally, ask yourself if you would enroll your family in the plan. If you don't feel comfortable in saying "yes", you may think twice about becoming a "participating provider."[121]

Another relationship issue has to do with continuity of care. Many managed care contracts contain clauses that permit them to "deselect" physicians at will, similar to the concept of "employment at will" which states that you may fire an employee at any time for any reason or no reason. A typical phrase: "Either party, with a ninety-day notice, may terminate this contract without cause." However, when these clauses are invoked, the patient relationship suffers.

Why would a health plan deselect a physician? Reasons vary. Health plans say decisions to drop individual doctors involve factors like board certification, geographic location, and patient satisfaction. Physicians often disagree, contending that health plans' actions are economically motivated, focusing on trends like the number of tests ordered or procedures performed. Adding to the physicians' anger is the fact that most plans don't publicize their selection and deselection criteria, or tell physicians what their utilization standards are. Further, under many contracts, there is no right of appeal.[122]

---

121 Ibid.,
122 *When healrh plans don't want you anymore.* Med Econ, May 23, 1994, p. 138-149.

Some managed care plans have continuity problems even when the patient's physician does participate. One doctor tells of a patient in New Mexico who may be admitted into the hospital for an emergency.[123] The staff physician on call admits the patient; later, another staff physician takes over and the patient may not see his or her regular physician for two or three days. Communication among all these physicians may be less than adequate. Excellent medical record documentation becomes critical; and if any of the physicians fails to document details, care could be seriously affected.

It is desirable to consider these tips:

Try to negotiate your contract. Admittedly this is difficult for solo practitioners, unless they're in great demand. However, groups can successfully negotiate changes in contract terminology. You may have better luck if you try negotiating with a plan that's new to town: it has a vested interest in signing up as many doctors as possible, and you have more leverage.[124]

Attempt to find out what standards are being used to judge you. Plans are notoriously resistant to sharing their criteria, but it has happened.

When you receive a new patient from the health plan, make sure the patient understands how long the relationship will last. For example, if you are a specialist receiving the patient on referral, let the patient know that when you release him, the relationship is over. Although this applies equally to traditional fee-for-service environments, m a managed care environment it is doubly important.

Finally, if you are in a private office environment (as opposed to an HMO clinic), make sure your staff members understand the importance of treating all patients with respect and dignity. Some staffers may consciously or unconsciously differentiate between private pay and managed care patients, treating the managed care patients as second-class citizens. It is critical that all patients be treated the same, in a caring, respectful manner.

---

123 *HMO crystallizes Albuquerque doctors 'fears.* Am Med News, July 25 1994, .p 19
124 Caesar NB. *How to gain leverage with a health plan.* Med Econ, February 7, 1994.

Cost-Based Risks

Earlier, we discussed some of the factors that make managed care attractive to those who seek to control health care costs. The reduction in inpatient days, the perception that plans deselect physicians who order too many tests and therefore cost more money - all of these present liability risks.

Chief of these is the very real issue of quality. If, in a physician's best medical judgment, a patient requires hospitalization and the authorization is denied, is the physician at risk? Similarly, if the patient is an ideal candidate for a drug in clinical trials but the plan refuses to pay, is the physician liable? What about the primary care doctor who knows his patient needs expert cardiac treatment, but the plan's participating physicians do not inspire confidence - could the primary care physician be liable if he refers his patient anyway?

By now, most physicians are aware of the landmark 1986 case Wickline vs. California.[125] Dr. Polansky performed two procedures on Lois Wickline, one to remove the left aorta and replace it with a Teflon graft, and another to remove a blood clot in her leg. Her recovery was troubled, and five days later she was returned to the OR where Dr. Polansky performed a lumbar sympathectomy. Medi-Cal had originally authorized a ten-day stay for the patient. Dr. Polansky sought an additional eight days as medically necessary, but Medicaal approved only four more days. Dr. Polansky acquiesced to Medical's decision. After discharge, Ms. Wickline developed complications and was readmitted, but the complications could not be remedied and her leg was amputated. She sued Medical and the state of California. Dr. Polansky, who was not a defendant, testified at trial that, if the additional four days had been approved, the deterioration would have been noticed and the amputation could have been prevented.

The case went to the California appellate court which ruled for the state. The court's reason: the physician had a responsibility to protest the decision of the third-party payer when that decision conflicted with the physician's medical judgment. To quote the court:

---

125 *Wickline v. California,* 183 Cal App 3rd 1175 (1986).

99

There is little doubt that Dr. Polansky was intimidated by the Medical program but he was not...powerless to act if other action was required... If, in his medical judgment, it was in his patient's best interest that she remain in the acute care hospital setting for an additional four days... Dr. Polansky should have made some effort to keep her there.

The warning is clear: if you disagree with the managed care plan's coverage decision, be prepared to fight.

How do you fight? Jason Collins, MD, an obstetrician who played a key role in another landmark managed care liability case, says the experience convinced him to document every element of every conversation with reviewers.[126] His case involved a pregnant woman whom he thought should be hospitalized during the last weeks of her pregnancy. United Healthcare, the Blue Cross utilization review company, refused to authorize the hospitalization, deciding that ten hours of home nursing care each day was the preferred course. Dr. Collins disagreed, but acquiesced. Thirteen days later, while Mrs. Corcoran was at home with no nurse present, the fetus went into distress and died.

The resulting malpractice suit alleged that United Healthcare and Blue Cross were at fault for failing to authorize the requested hospitalization. The case went to the Fifth Circuit Court of Appeals, which heard the defense argue that United Healthcare was simply interpreting benefits. According to defense attorneys, Mrs. Corcoran could have opted for hospitalization anyway, paying for it out of her pocket. The plaintiffs argued that was absurd: the point of insurance is to protect people from bankruptcy, not force them into it. The court took the middle ground: it held that utilization review companies make medical decisions incidental to benefit determinations, noting that, when benefit determinations are made prior to treatment, the firms are making medical recommendations which, because of the financial ramifications, are more likely to be followed.[127]

---

126 *Courts support health insurers that reject "unnecessa,y" care.* Wall St. Journal, November 25, 1992, p. B-8
127 Azevedo O. *Courts let UR firms off the hook-and leave doctors on.* Med Econ, January 25, 1993., p. 30-44.

Other risks involve denial of payment for treatments deemed "experimental" by UR or managed care organizations. The 1993 case Fox v. HealthNet illustrates how denial can backfire for the managed care organization.[128] HealthNet, a California HMO, refused to authorize payment for autologous bone marrow transplants for Nelene Fox, a 37-year-old patient with breast cancer. The HMO asserted that such treatments were experimental, despite opinions from several noted oncologists who held that the transplants were accepted therapy. The patient raised the money, though it took six months. She ended up paying for the transplants herself, and ultimately died. Her estate sued the HMO, and a jury agreed that the HMO was negligent in failing to authorize payment for the treatment, stating that the six-month delay contributed to the patient's death. Damages totaled 89 million dollars, reflecting the jury's anger at the arbitrary, financially motivated decision of the HMO. As a result, other HMOs and insurers have changed their policies.[129]

In addition to Dr. Collins' tip about documenting every detail of every conversation you have with the managed care organization or UR firm, the following suggestions are offered:[130]

Get the caller's full name and title or identification number and the company's name. Also get the name of the insured arrangement they work for (if they don't work directly for the insurer) and the group or certificate number of the patient. If they can't or won't provide this information, don't give them medical information.

Be sure you're actually dealing with a person or entity authorized to receive this confidential information. As noted above, get the caller's full identification, then consider calling back to make sure the phone is answered appropriately. With the new privacy rules set forth by the Health Insurance Portability and Accountability Act (HIP AA), this is doubly important.

You usually don't need a signed release from your patient. Patients sign such authorizations when they join the managed care plan. However, you can always request a copy of the authorization for your files.

---

128 *Fox v. Health Net of Cal.,* No. 219692, Ca. Super. Ct. (Riverside) (1993.)
129 Anders G. *More insurers pay for care that's in trials.* Wall St. Journal, February 15, 1994, p. 8-1
130 Dabbs M. *Take the offensive: tips for handling utilization review.* Tex Med, March, 1991, p. 60-61

Consider recording the conversation with the reviewer, stating that your motive is to make sure there's no misunderstanding regarding your intent to provide the best possible patient care. If they refuse to talk to you on that basis, document the refusal and the date.

Don't let reviewers take you away from patient care. Tell them you will call back when you are not busy with patients and ask for a toll free number if they have one.

Don't talk with them until you are familiar with the patient and treatment plan. Make sure you review the record before you get on the phone.

Give reviewers only basic information directly related to the need for hospitalization or continued stay. If they ask for more details, ask to speak to a physician or tell them the requested information is not necessary.

If you are talking to a non-physician who doesn't seem to understand the patient's condition, ask to speak with a supervisor or a physician.

Don't let non-physicans make final decisions to deny payment. Insist on speaking to a physician.

Don't provide sensitive information like HIV status or psychiatric or substance abuse information without written authorization from the patient. This will help you comply with HIPAA privacy regulations and state regulations.

Document all contact, including times you called but got no answer, or were on hold for excessive periods. If you are put on hold for longer than seems reasonable, hang up, document the attempted contact and call back at your convenience.

Work in concert with your hospital's UR department. Often, they are more knowledgeable about specific firms.

If payment is denied:

Ask why. Try to get the criteria used. Sometimes this information will be provided.

Request a retrospective review from the review company.

Send written protests or appeals to the review company and send copies of your letters to the patient. Assist your patient in appealing as well.

Let your patient know about the consequences of not continuing with the treatment. If the patient decides not to continue treatment, document that decision and the reason. It helps if your patient will sign an informed refusal statement.

Consider bypassing the UR firm and going directly to the insurance company. Let the insurer know they are responsible for the acts of their agents, including the UR company. Send copies to all concerned parties, including the patient.

Most of all, remember that if you do what's right for the patient, you will be judged more compassionately by a jury than if you give in to what the UR and managed care organizations say.

Liability for MCOs and Physicians

If you participate in a managed care plan and you're sued for malpractice, is your liability different from what it is under traditional fee-for-service?

The answer: perhaps. It will depend on the nature of the managed care organization, your contract, whether the managed care organization is covered by ERISA, and the nature of the allegations.

The Nature of the Managed Care Organization

Staff model HMOs, which directly employ physicians, have always been held liable in negligence cases under the vicarious liability theory of respondeat superior, much as a hospital would be liable for its employed nurses and therapists. The key is control: if it can be demonstrated that the organization controls the actions of its employees, then the organization has liability for the actions of its employees.[131]

---

131 *Sloan v. Metropolitan Health Council,* 516 .E.2nd 1104 (Ind. Cl. of App. 1987 .).

However, group and IPA model HMOs are different from staff model HMOs. With group and IPA models, the HMO contracts with independent physicians to provide health care services, and it may be argued that the HMO does not control these independent contractors. Seven criteria are used to determine whether or not a physician is an independent contractor, including such factors as the right of control over performance, the method of payment, manner of selection and engagement, and ownership of facilities used to perform the work.[132] If the physician can be shown to be a truly independent contractor, chances are the HMO would have no liability for the physician's actions.[133]

The liability described above is clear: a physician who works for or contracts with an HMO that exercises certain control over the physician's actions will, for the purposes of tort liability, be considered an actual agent of the managed care organization. Therefore, if there is a claim of malpractice, the physician will be sued and the managed care organization may be sued as well, subject to ERISA preemption, as discussed later.

What about a physician who really is an independent contractor? Does that automatically mean he or she will bear the full burden of any suit filed (i.e., would the managed care organization be excluded?) Not necessarily. There is another theory of liability, called ostensible or apparent agency, which is concerned with whether or not the physician appears to be an agent of the HMO. For example, if the patient considers himself to be a patient of the HMO rather than of Dr. X, and/or if the HMO "holds out" the doctor as being its employee, then there could be made a case for ostensible agency.

Key points:

Does the patient have a choice in selection of his or her physician? If not, then it could be said that the patient "looked to the institution" for care, and the doctor was an ostensible agent of the managed care organization.

---

132 Restatement (Second) of Agency § 220 (1958.).
I 33 Chittenden, *supra*

Does the organization "hold out" the physician to be its employee? In other words, if the physician is identified with the HMO on billing, correspondence, medical releases and similar documents, then it could be said that the doctor was the ostensible agent of the HMO. For IPA arrangements, however, courts have held that the HMO does not "hold itself out" to be a health care provider, and since it doesn't fall under the definition of a "health care provider," it cannot practice medicine, and therefore cannot be held liable in and of itself.[134]

Both *respondeat superior* and ostensible agency fall under the legal theory of vicarious liability, meaning that liability is imposed on one person or entity for the actionable conduct of another. A physician is vicariously liable for the actions of his employees, just as the HMO could be held vicariously liable for the actions of its employed or contracted physicians, under the scenarios so briefly described.

However, there are other types of liability. Direct liability may also fall upon the HMO for negligent selection of physician staff, negligent supervision or control of physician actions, and such "alternative" theories of liability as breach of warranty, breach of contract, and fraud. How Managed Care Organizations Defend Themselves

The purpose of this chapter is to orient physician readers to types of managed care liabilities and ways to counter them, not to teach them the law. However, there are some important points regarding managed care liability that physicians should know. ERISA (the Employee Retirement Income Security Act of 1974) was designed to protect pension plans but now affects nearly two-thirds of all employee health benefit plans. The definition of an employee welfare benefit plan is broad, but includes any plan or program established by an employer for the purpose of providing medical care or benefits to its employees through the purchase of insurance or by other means.[135] Managed care programs established through contract with an HMO, PPO or standard insurer meet that definition and may therefore be covered under ERIS A. By law, ERISA supersedes state laws governing how benefits are handled.

---

134 *Picket v. CIGNA Healthplan Services, Inc.* No. 01/92/00803/CV, Tex. App. - Hjuston (1ˢᵗ District], 17 June 1993., writ rejected), 1993. WL 209858.
135 Chittendon, supra, p. 485.

Therefore, if a malpractice case is brought against an HMO, and there is clear evidence of negligence, causation and damages, but the HMO is contracted by a benefits plan run by a self-insured company for the benefit of its employees, then typically £RISA would prevail and the HMO may not be sued, despite the existence of negligence. It is on the basis of £RISA that the Corcorans in Corcoran v. United Health Care were barred from suing.[136] It is also on that basis that the American Medical Association has called for changes in £RISA, to hold managed care plans accountable for their decisions.

In light of £RISA, is it possible that malpractice lawsuits against insurance plans will be allowed to proceed? To some extent, yes. The £RISA preemption is eroding slightly on a case-by-case basis. The majority of states allow some form of litigation against insurance plans that are covered by £RISA. Many of the lawsuits that have been decided in favor of plaintiffs are under appeal, so the final tally is subject to change.

Tips for Managing Managed Care Risks

If you are sued for malpractice by a plaintiff covered by a managed care contract, the plaintiffs attorney may seek a link between you and the HMO. Why? The HMO, like the physician, will have liability insurance; and if the plaintiff can tap into those "deep pockets", the damages may be greatly increased.

To create that link, the plaintiffs attorney is going to scrutinize the contracts linking the physician to the HMO. He or she will search for clauses regarding duration of contract, payment for physician services, procedures to follow if there is disagreement about professional services - in short, anything that will bolster the claim that the defendant physician was the direct or ostensible agent of the HMO.

---

136 *Corcoran v. United Healthcare,* supra.

Clauses and phrases to watch out for:

Indemnification clauses, which state that you are solely responsible for the medical management of the patient. Such clauses will put you at full risk if there's a problem with the patient's care, even if you're just following treatment decisions made by utilization reviewers. These clauses would cause you to pay all judgments against the HMO when it's named in a suit along with you. Some contracts even require physicians to hold the managed care organization harmless from all liability, even legal liability for their decisions to deny care or payment for care.[137]

Clauses which cause you to comply with a utilization review plan or quality assurance plan. These plans are set by the managed care organization, not you. They could change tomorrow, and you would still be bound by them.

Clauses which force you to refer only to other member physicians. If you refer a patient to a specialist on the panel, but that specialist bungles the case, you could be held liable for negligent referral, even though the plan gave you no choice.

You also should discuss legal risks accrued to the physician. Many plans don't have their own professional liability insurance, and try to piggyback their risks onto the doctor. Therefore, you should check to make sure that the plan does have insurance. Otherwise, be especially careful of the indemnification clauses.

What can you do to protect yourself against these new managed care risks? As with traditional fee-for-service medicine, practicing exemplary medicine is no guarantee that you won't be sued. So, you need to be prepared.

Review the proposed contract carefully. Get an attorney skilled m health care law to work with you. Together, check the contract for:

Indemnification clauses (the "hold harmless" clauses mentioned above). If they are present, check with your insurer to see if you would still be covered if you signed the agreement. Or, refuse to sign. Or, insist on a mutual indemnification clause. You have choices; don't automatically accept the clause just because it's there.

---

137 Keddie-Holt J. *Managed care: recognizing and managing professional liability risks.* TMLT Reporter, Vol. 12, No. 3

Requirements about liability insurance. The plan should require all physicians to carry adequate malpractice insurance. Otherwise, if you were named as codefendant in a case principally focusing on another HMO physician, and that doctor didn't carry insurance, in some states you could be held liable for the entire damage award.

Remember that if all malpractice insurers were to be required to provide essentially "full" coverage to managed care plans, the cost of your malpractice insurance may skyrocket.

Peer review and credentialing procedures. These criteria determine the caliber of physicians in the panel. If there are loose or unenforced criteria, you may be practicing with physicians to whom you'd rather not refer or be associated with.

Look for plans that are patient-friendly. If the plan would require you to accept more patients than you feel appropriate, insist that the quota be changed. Lack of time to examine and treat patients is a leading cause, of suits alleging failure to diagnose, delay in treatment, etc. Make sure the plan doesn't burden you with more than you can handle. Resist the temptation to double the patient load for half the capitation fee.

Study case #1

A patient who was covered by an HMO had cardiac problems. The HMO represented that ongoing care by the patient's own physician would be covered, but later denied such coverage. The HMO also did not issue the patient an ID card which resulted in delay in care by his primary physician. When the patient finally got in to see his own physician, that doctor said he didn't know anything about the HMO's procedure for referrals to specialists. Finally, the HMO allegedly prevented the patient from obtaining medication. by providing erroneous information to a pharmacy. When the patient died of his cardiac problem, the family sued the HMO, its medical director and the private care physician, based on breach of contract, misrepresentation, breach of fiduciary duty, negligence, medical malpractice, professional misconduct and negligent infliction of emotional distress. The HMO and the medical director moved for dismissal on grounds that the state law claims as set forth were preempted by ERISA.[138]

---

138 *Nealy v. U.S. Health Care HMO,* 844 F.Supp. 966 (S.D .. Y. 1994)

Do you think the HMO was negligent?

What about the medical director?

Was the private physician negligent?

Do you think that the suit will survive ERISA?

See below for discussion.

Discussion

If the facts are as stated, the HMO would seem negligent. It should have stuck by its promise to pay for the patient to see his private physician; it should have made sure the patient had an ID card if that's what it took to get care; it should have made sure the private physician knew about the HMO's policies regarding referrals outside the panel; and it should have facilitated the patient's prescription. It apparently did none of these. The medical director was responsible for the HMO's medical decisions and he never saw the patient. Further, he was involved in administrative decisions, not just clinical decisions. There was no evidence that he was personally involved with the decisions regarding this patient's care. Therefore, the court dismissed him from the case.

The private physician did not join in the motion for dismissal. The court proceeded to find that the medical malpractice claim against him was not subject to dismissal. The reason: the physician's direct provision of medical treatment did not relate to the health plan.

Note: This is a good example of how managed care problems affect physician liability. It's obvious that the plan was negligent in failing to provide the patient with needed documentation and information. The physician, in attempting to adhere to the plan's rules, did not treat the patient on a timely basis. However, when the suit was filed, the plan argued that it should be dropped from the suit because of ERISA. When the court agreed, the private physician was left holding the bag.

If a private physician contracts with an HMO to become a "health care provider," he or she should be prepared to take extra steps to assure that care is provided in a timely manner. The Nealy case illustrates that when plans make mistakes, the patient suffers. And, in the long run, it's the doctor, not the plan, who is most frequently held liable.

6. PSYCHOLOGIC UNDERSTANDING AND MANAGEMENT OF THE PLASTIC SURGERY PATIENTS

Mastering the art of plastic surgery requires a deep appreciation of the degree to which physical appearance affects self-concept and wellbeing. Understanding and managing the psychologic concerns of plastic surgery patients is essential for problem prevention, including reducing the likelihood of patient dissatisfaction and malpractice litigation. More important, this understanding facilitates achieving the primary mission of plastic surgery - maximizing patient quality of life. If surgeons steadily develop their skills in understanding patients' psychologic concerns, they and their patients will be richly rewarded with the fruits of the "magic" of plastic surgery - the ability to change patients' psyche in a positive way by improving their appearance.[139]

This chapter describes the information and skills plastic surgeons need to understand and manage patient psychological concerns by addressing three topics:

Defining body image and describing how it is central to understanding the motivations for, and impact of, plastic surgery. Reviewing critical psychologic issues in cosmetic surgery, including assessing patient expectations, screening for psychopathology, insuring informed consent and evaluating postoperative psychologic responses to surgery. Reviewing critical factors in treating patients undergoing reconstructive surgery, including: describing patterns of psychologic response to reconstructive surgery; suggesting constructive methods of patient referral for psychiatric evaluation and treatment; defining factors influencing patient response to disfigurement; and advocating for the use of all available resources to maximize psychologic rehabilitation.

---

139 Jonathan M. Sykes/ Managing the psychological aspects of plastic surgery patients, 2009.

Body Image and Plastic Surgery

The ultimate goal of plastic surgery is to alter the patient's body image (i.e., to change their subjective perception of their body and to improve the patient's quality of life). To fully understand the power, beauty, and "magic" of plastic surgery, and to be effective in managing the psychologic concerns of patients, the surgeon must understand body image.[140]

A critical facet of body image is the degree to which it is directly related to feelings about self. Stated simply, if we feel positive about our bodies, we are more likely to feel positively about ourselves and our lives. The most important disease treated by plastic surgeons is the feelings associated with deformity (8), including a sense of personal inadequacy that strikes at the heart of identity - the sense of self.

Robert Goldwyn reminds us that the word *patient* is derived from *patient*, Latin for "to suffer" and that suffering is not confined to physical pain and loss of function, for plastic surgery patients, suffering is largely the result of a negative body image. The plastic surgeon's professional mission is to relieve this suffering by facilitating the patient's creation of a more positive body image.[141]

CHANGING NEGATIVE BODY IMAGE

Psychologic changes brought about by plastic surgery focus on reducing the negative feelings an individual has about physical appearance. Specifically, plastic surgery facilitates changes in body-image cognition, emotion, and behavior.[142]

---

140 Jonathan M. ykes / Managing the psychological aspects of plastic surgery patients, 2009.
141 Randy A. Sam one MD, Lori A. Sam one MD/ Cosmetic surgery and psychological issue , Psychiatry (Edgmont), 2007.
142 Ibid.

Body Image Cognition

Body-image cognition refers to the thinking that all individuals engage in regarding their appearance. These cognitive processes may include self-talk (e.g., "My nose is really ugly"), images (pictures the patient has of self-appearance in own mind), or beliefs about appearance (e.g., "If I am disfigured [have small breasts, etc.], then I cannot be happy"). If surgery results in positive changes in appearance, individuals can then begin to think differently about themselves (i.e., change the way they talk to, imagine or believe in themselves). However, the surgical change in appearance must be positive in the eyes or the patient.

Body image is, by definition, subjective. You cannot know how someone feels about their body on the basis o evaluating their objective appearance. This point is central to understanding and managing all plastic surgery patients: *Perception of appearance is completely subjective, and changes in appearance are "improvements" only if the patient evaluates them as such.*

Body Image Emotions

Negative thinking patterns (or their positive and adaptive counterparts) can dramatically influence emotions. Consistently engaging in self-talk that is derogatory (e.g .. "My nose is disgusting"), having a visual image of myself as "ugly" and believing that I am unlovable, my emotions will be directly affected. Depending upon the situation, I may become depressed, resigned, angry, or anxious as a result of this pattern of thinking. Current psychologic techniques can change negative patterns of thinking regarding one's body, which can lead to change in negative patterns of feeling.[143]

---

143 Randy A. Samsone MD, Lori A. Samsone MD / Cosmetic surgery and psychological issues, Psychiatry (Edgmont), 2007.

Body Image Behavior

Patterns of negative thinking and emotion are invariably associated with patterns of maladaptive behavior. Patients who think they are ugly, and who feel ashamed of their appearance, are likely to develop negative patterns of social interaction (e.g., social withdrawal). Many levels of social interaction can be affected by negative patterns of body image cognition and emotions, including nonverbal behavior during everyday communication and sexual functioning. For example, women with breast disfigurement may believe that "I am not attractive to my partner," feel ashamed of their appearance, and therefore avoid any kind of sexual contact. Positive changes in patterns of thinking can set the stage for, and be facilitated by, positive changes in behavior (e.g., increased positive social interaction).[144]

SUMMARY

The motivation to undergo plastic surgery is a sense of disease and body image discomfort that strikes at the heart of an individual's sense of identity. Fully understanding the motivations for and the effects of plastic surgery requires insight into how the individual's subjective perception of his body affects his thinking, emotion, and behavior. By creating changes in physical appearance the patient perceives as positive, surgeons set the stage for patients to change their patterns of thinking, emotion, and behavior. Most important, they have helped individuals to change their identity and overall quality of life.

Cosmetic Surgery Patients: Psychologic Issues

The critical variables essential to understanding and caring for the psychologic needs of cosmetic surgery patients include: (a) understanding patient expectations, (h) screening for the most common common forms of psychopathology, (c) assessing patients' evaluation of surgical risk tied benefit, and (d) evaluating the postoperative psychologic impact of surgery.[145] All four sets of variables are essential to consider. Shortcuts for the sake of clinical efficiency are possible, but only at the cost of compromising clinical effectiveness.

---

144 Ibid.
145 Ibid.,

ASSESSING PATIENT EXPECTATIONS

Cosmetic surgery patients have three distinct types of expectations. They obviously have expectations regarding the desired changes in appearance. Additionally, they have explicit or implicit expectations regarding how they will respond emotionally to surgery (i.e. psychologic expectations) and how others will respond to them (i.e. social expectations).

Understanding all three sets of expectations serves to structure preoperative patient evaluation. The relevant information can be elicited relatively quickly and with little intrusiveness. Failure to evaluate any of these expectations increases the likelihood of patient dissatisfaction. By evaluating expectations, the surgeon conveys concern tor the patient's total well-being, thus laying a solid foundation for the development of a positive professional relationship. There is nothing in more fundamental to psychologic understanding and managing patients than paying close and constant attention to the patient-physician relationship.

Surgical Expectations

It is imperative that patients have clear and realistic expectations regarding the surgical changes they desire. The ability to distinguish between "realistic" and "idealistic" expectations regarding surgical outcome is highly predictive of patient satisfaction with surgical outcome. Recent research strongly suggests that idealistic expectations are pathognomonic of potential problems postoperatively. Additionally, creating high patient expectations through advertising or by compiling "a flattering portfolio of excellent results for prospective patients to review" risks increasing the probability of some patients being disappointed postoperatively.[146]

---

146 Randy A. Samsone MD, Lori A. Samsone MD I Cosmetic surgery and psychological is ues, Psychiatry (Edgmont), 2007.

Fundamental and seemingly obvious principle of psychologic management is that the patient's subjective evaluation of the surgical outcome determines the ultimate impact of cosmetic surgery (i.e., the degree to which the patient's quality of life is improved). This fundamental observation leads to the admonition against surgeons imposing their own aesthetic standards on patients. The surgeon must view the outcome of the operation through the eyes of the patient, not from the perspective of objective aesthetic standards or the surgeon's subjective perception. It is the patient's subjective perception of the surgical outcome that is the gold standard by which the success of surgery is measured.[147]

We were reminded of this fundamental principle recently when evaluating a male patient who underwent rhinoplasty for a posttraumatic deformity (to straighten the nose) but who did not expect a reduction in the dorsal hump. At the time of the initial preoperative consultation there was only a brief discussion of the hump reduction (which was undertaken) and an extended discussion of chin augmentation (which the patient did not request, want, or undergo). The patient was partly dissatisfied with the postoperative nasal appearance. In this instance, the surgeon undertook the "reasonable" (but wrong) approach of reducing the prominent hump "while he was there"; however, this was not in keeping with the patient's expectations. The patient was pleased with the postoperative nasal straightening but not with nasal reduction.

Positive changes in appearance are defined as "positive" by the pattern. Suggestions for surgical improvements not requested by the patient (e.g., those offered by the surgeon or family members) should be undertaken with only the greatest of care, if at all, and only after multiple preoperative evaluations. Additionally, patients who have vague nonspecific requests for surgical change, or those willing to defer the definition of change to the surgeon, should be approached with great caution.

---

147 Ibid.

116

Psychologic Expectations

All patients seeking cosmetic surgery arc motivated to change their body image (i.e., to change the psychologic experience of their body and achieve a reduction in body-image dysphoria). Having obtained a clear understanding of surgical expectations, and assuming these are reasonable, the surgeon should make a statement similar to the following: "All of my patients have hopes about how they are going to feel after surgery. How do you imagine you will feel after undergoing the operation? We know surgery can change how you look, but how do you think the operation might change your life?"

Many patients will respond with a reply similar to the following: "l will feel better about myself." The surgeon should inquire further about the nature of the motivations and emotions leading up to the request for surgery. For example, the surgeon can ask: "How has your appearance affected the way you feel about yourself?" "How long have you been thinking about having surgery?" "When did you first start to think about if?" "Why do you want surgery now and not a year ago or a year in the future?" "In what way has your appearance affected your behavior?" "How do you expect to feel, think or act differently after surgery?" "In what specific situations do you believe you will be more comfortable after having the operation?"

Answers to such questions provide the surgeon with some of the information necessary to ascertain if the patient has reasonable expectations. Even more important, such questions provide insight into the patient's overall psychologic motioning and may reveal any current or past psychopathology.

Social Expectations

To understand the patient's social expectations, it is helpful to know how the individuals closest to the patient feel about the operation. How does the patient expect the important people in his life will respond to the operation? Are they supportive? Are they in any way responsible for the patient wanting the surgery? If a patient is being "pushed" by a family member, or if a patient is going against the advice of a close family member, these factors can significantly influence the patient's ultimate reaction to the operation. Preoperative discussion of these issues can be productive, particularly if the patient is hoping to change the behavior of someone else as a result of undergoing surgery (e.g., to win someone's affection).[148]

Summary

Any indication at patient expectations regarding the surgical, psychologic, or social outcome of surgery are problematic and warrant a more intensive patient evaluation. In many instances, surgeons may want to insure clear communication regarding expectations by routinely scheduling multiple preoperative, patient evaluations. In some instances, the psychologic safety and efficacy of providing surgery may be questioned. In those instances, a more complete psychologic evaluation is required.

SCREENING FOR PSYCHOLOGIC DISORDERS

Most cosmetic surgery patients do not evidence psychopathology. However, a significant minority present with some form of psychologic disorder that requires a more complete psychologic evaluation and that may affect the decision to undertake surgery. Disorders that may be encountered include: Body Dysmorphic Disorder, Personality Disorders and eating Disorders (DSM-1 V). Other psychologic problems encountered in cosmetic surgery patients include depression, alcohol abuse, and anxiety. These will be reviewed later.

---

148 Altamura C. Paluello MO, Clinical and subclinical body dismorphic disorder, Eur Arch Psychiatry Clinic neuroscience, 2001.

Body Dysmorphic Disorder (BDD)

Patients with Body Dysmorphic Disorder (HDD) are well known to plastic surgeons. The defining feature of BDD is that the patient has an intensely negative emotional response to some aspect of their appearance, despite the fact that there is little or no evidence for objective deformity. These patients often present with the classic contraindications for cosmetic surgery, including minimal deformity, multiple consultations with plastic surgeons, the obsessive focus on appearance and emotional volatility.[149]

Currently, there are no accurate estimates of the incidence of BDD in the population of cosmetic surgery patients. Additionaly, the intensity of symptom presentation is widely variable. A subgroup of patients appear to have psychotic features, making the differential diagnosis of BDD from somatic delusions critical to consider.

BDD patients arc invariably challenging to the surgeon and require special management and tremendous amounts of consultation time. Psychiatric input into the evaluation and possible treatment of BDD patients is absolutely necessary. The challenge of differential diagnosis (e.g. psychotic versus non psychotic symptom presentation), issues of patient impotency to make medical decisions and to provide informed consent, possible alternative or adjunctive approaches in treatment, and predictions regarding the safety and efficacy of undertaking surgery with these patients are all areas in which the psychiatric consultation is mandatory.

Many surgeons choose to eliminate these patients from their practices, believing that they cannot be helped with surgery, and lacking experience in treating such patients. However, extensive clinical experience has demonstrated that many individuals with similar symptoms can be helped with a well-structured program of surgicalpsychologic evaluation and intervention. The resources to conduct such programs are not widely available, and there are some important differences of opinion regarding treatment strategics and efficacy. However, plastic surgeons have a professional obligation to address the needs of these long-suffering patients.

---

149 Ibid.,

Personality Disorders

Experienced observers of the psychologic functioning of plastic surgery patients have described specific and unique patterns of maladaptive patient responses to stress. Napoleon identified the most common personality types observed in plastic surgery, including patients with narcissistic, dependent and borderline personality features.[150]

Patients with narcissistic personalities are among the most common in plastic surgery. In addition to being arrogant, the have a grandiose sense of self-importance and a belief they are special, and they also feel entitled to special treatment. Their hypersensitivity to any social slight, fragile self-esteem, and belief that there should be automatic compliance with their expectations, places them at increased risk for negative responses to even minor problems (e.g., small complications, brief delays). They arc more likely to seek legal recourse for the "wrongs" that have been done to them. When their very strong needs for approval and praise are unfulfilled, patient management problems ensue. These patients must be handled with special care, because they respond negatively to any perceived slight.

However, patients with dependent personality are usually passive individuals who look to other people to make their decisions, take responsibility for them, and to provide reassurance. They are often very reluctant to express their real feelings and thoughts because of their desperate need to obtain the approval of others. "When all is going well such people are amiable, obliging, and a pleasure to be around." However, they are at increased risk for postoperative disappointment if they do not clearly express their expectations for the outcome of surgery. Additionally, under the stress of surgery they can become very "needy," demanding, and childlike, sometimes alternating between angry outbursts (often directed at support staff) and tearful apologies (to the surgeon). "They require expressions of warmth and concern."

---

150 Jonathan M. Sykes/ Managing the psychological aspects of plastic surgery patients, 2009.

Plastic surgery patients with borderline personality characteristics are among the most challenging to manage. By definition, these individuals are emotionally volatile, unstable, and impulsive. This personality type is likely to be the least satisfied with surgery. Additionally, for these individuals, even small complications can result in "a catastrophe of immense proportions."[151] It also appears that they are more likely to initiate legal action. Of greatest clinical relevance to their management is that patients with borderline personality features often enter into the patient-physician relationship with an extremely positive (albeit inflated) evaluation of the surgeon. The scenario patient idealization is a theme that is evident when analyzing the dynamics of plastic surgery malpractice claims.

Characteristically, the initial patient-surgeon contact had been one where the surgeon was idealized in the eyes of the patient. In each case, this idealization transformed into hatred postoperatively. The transformation from "all good" to "all bad" had begun, but was not "caused," by a postoperative medical complication in each malpractice claim. Idealization, therefore, can be an early warning of the problems to come.[152]

Therefore, surgeons should be even more cautious when encountering patients who place them on a "pedestal." This idealization may indicate inflated and unachievable expectations (regarding all aspects of care) and may indicate the presence of borderline personality disorder.

151 Ahamura C. Paluello MD, Clinical and ubclinical body dismorphic disorder, Eur Arch Psychiatry Clinic neuroscience, 2001.
152 Jonathan M. Syke / Managing the psychological a peels ofpla tic surgery patients, 2009.

Evaluating patient personality functioning is very challenging. It is most effectively accomplished by monitoring the patient-surgeon relationship. Clues to predicting patient management problems are often evident on the basis of how the patient makes the surgeon feel. If the surgeon begins to feel irritated, angry, or uncomfortable, or if the surgeon has an atypical emotional response to a patient, this can be an important stimulus to "step back" and scrutinize the patient's psychologic functioning. Additionally, the physician should play close attention to the emotional reactions of trusted staff members to specific patients. Individuals with personality disorders often elicit conflict among staff members who ordinarily interact well together. In general, if a patient is eliciting significant negative attention from those involved in their care, this is an important clue to devote even greater amounts of time and attention to psychologic issues.

Eating Disorders

As many as 8% of the female adolescent and young adult population in the United States have some symptoms of Anorexia Nervosa and/or Bulimia Nervosa. These young women are preoccupied with their physical appearance and experience body image distortions. They engage in dieting and extreme forms of appetite and weight control. As a general rule, they take great efforts to keep their symptoms hidden.[153]

Some of these individuals seek out plastic surgery and are most likely to request body sculpting procedures, liposuction and breast related operations. Some patients may request changes in facial appearance (e.g., reduction of enlarged parotid glands).

The problem with providing these young women with surgery is that the procedures only addresses a symptom of a much larger problem with body dissatisfaction and distortion. Though they are likely to be pleased with the surgical outcome, it is not clear that surgery results in an overall improvement in quality of life or a fundamental change in body image. When surgeons suspect that a young woman requesting surgery may have an eating disorder, they should directly address their concern.

---

153 Altamura C. Paluello MD, Clinical and subclinical body dismorphic disorder, Eur Arch P ychiatry Clinic neuroscience, 2001.

EVALUATING PATIENT PERCEPTION OF SURGICAL RISK AND BENEFIT

The primary reason to undertake the risks inherent in any surgical procedure is the physical and psychologic benefit of the operation. "The weighing of risks and benefits for cosmetic surgery is directly related to the patient's psychologic expectations for cosmetic surgery, and therefore, in effect, it is a requirement of the informed consent process to discuss these expectations."[154]

Therefore, in the initial evaluation of cosmetic surgery patients, it is essential to review their evaluation of surgical risk and benefit. How well does the patient under-stand and remember the explanation of the risks described by the surgeon, and how does he weigh these in comparison to the expected benefits of surgery? The surgeon must focus on the risks of surgery (including postoperative discomfort, risk of minor and serious complications, changes in sensory functioning, and the permanent impact of surgical scars) and how these are evaluated in relation to the expected benefits.

SUMMARY

Remember that the only indication for cosmetic surgery is to improve emotional health. Thus, effective management of cosmetic surgery patients requires that attention be given to psychologic factors. In addition to the patient types already described, some others require extra attention, including women desiring removal of breast implants, adolescents and persons who are potentially somewhat more psychologically vulnerable than the typical cosmetic surgery patient.

Furthermore, attention given to psychologic factors should extend to evaluating patient response in the postoperative period. Inevitably, there are a minority of patients who are dissatisfied with a less-than-ideal surgical outcome. If given the full attention they feel they deserve, and if there arc no violations of their expectations, they will respond positively to the surgery.

---

154 Randy A. Sam one MD, Lori A. Sam one MD I Cosmetic surgery and psychological issue , Psychiatry (Edgmont), 2007.

In this situation, the wise advice of Robert Goldwyn should be followed, that is, admit the reality, make a very clear plan for addressing the problem, enlist the patient's support and be sure that you are readily available to the patient.[155]

For those patients who are dissatisfied despite a technically successful surgery, retrospective analysis often reveals that some of the factors already discussed (e.g., violations of implicit or explicit expectations or patient psychopathology) resulted in the patient dissatisfaction. These patients should receive a great deal of attention and be given appointments at times when the surgeon will not be rushed and can devote their full attention to the patient The surgeon must resist the natural tendency to withdraw emotionally from these individuals. In some instances, a surgical and/or psychiatric consultant will be of great help in addressing patient concerns.

Reconstructive Surgery Patients: Critical Psychologic Issues

Plastic surgeons contribute to the psychologic adaptation of reconstructive surgery patients by adapting their professional style of interaction to the patient's particular emotional response, identifying problematic psychologic responses and, when necessary, providing compelling and compassionate referral for psychiatric evaluation and treatment Patients greatly appreciate surgeons taking a genuine interest in their psychosocial functioning in addition to minimizing disfigurement and maximizing function.

GENERAL PRINCIPLES OF PSYCHOLOGICAL MANAGEMENT

Some helpful general principles for managing the psychologic concerns of reconstructive surgery patients include the following:

Ideally, surgeons assist patients and families in creating realistic expectations for the process and outcome of surgical reconstruction in the most consistent and compassionate manner possible. The surgeon's challenge is to maintain the delicate balance between hope and surgical reality.

---

155 Ibid.

Describing the process and outcome of surgical reconstruction is beyond the task of obtaining informed consent for any specific procedure. Rather, repeated and accurate description of the final surgical outcome (to the degree this is possible) and the entire process of surgical reconstruction is essential to striking the balance between hope and reality.

The difficulties and shortcomings of the reconstruction must be discussed when patients can assimilate the information, and with language the family understands. Repeating information may be necessary, and will cultivate the trust and understanding essential to establishing the patient-physician relationship.

The most powerful step in establishing the patient-physician professional relationship is to follow a basic rule for highly effective human relations: "Seek first to understand and only then to be understood." Surgeons are advised to practice the seemingly obvious principle of seeking first to understand clearly each patient's unique concerns before providing information or reassurance. "Facile, nonspecific reassurance can undermine the physician-patient relationship as the patient is likely to feel the physician is out of touch with and not really interested in what they are actually feeling."

The plastic surgeon can significantly enhance their ability to care for patients by learning to identify and effectively respond to the most common patterns of psychologic reactions-including anxiety, depression, and substance abuse, as well as denial and regression.

Surgeons can develop effective responses to these patient reactions. Depending on the particular situation, the surgeon can provide an increased level of psychologic support, treat the symptoms of emotional distress, or refer the patient for psychiatric evaluation and treatment.

How surgeons refer patients for psychiatric consultation dramatically influences patient compliance with the recommendation. A critical step toward creating a convincing, and compassionate referral for psychiatric evaluation (for constructive and cosmetic surgery) is for the surgeon to have complete confidence in the psychiatrist's ability to provide services tailored to plastic surgery patients.

To complete this prerequisite, surgeons should establish a long-term relationship with a psychiatric consultant who will evaluate the full spectrum of plastic surgery patients and who is familiar with the professional literature on the psychologic aspects of plastic surgery. Taking these steps will reduce the discomfort shared by many surgeons in commending psychiatric evaluation to patients.

In general, it is most helpful to establish a relationship with a psychiatrist (as opposed to a clinical psychologist or clinical social worker) because of the need for the consultant to evaluate the patient's medical history, the possible role medications in causing or exacerbating psycho logic symptoms, and if necessary, to prescribe psychotropic medications.

When surgeons refer patients for psychiatric evaluation, they should do so "... with the same attitude and for the same reasons as in the referral to, for example, a cardiologist". The surgeon can explain exactly why the referral is needed and not fumble around or use euphemisms such as "nerve doctor" or "another specialist". "Call the psychiatrist a psychiatrist." It is also essential to convey to the patient that you are doing what you believe to be in their best interests. Remind the patient that all deformities cause some emotional distress and some problems in adaptation.

PSYCHOLOGIC RESPONSE TO DISFIGUREMENT AND SURGICAL RECONSTRUCTION

Plastic surgeons regularly encounter predictable patterns of psychologic response to disfigurement and surgical reconstruction, including (a) anxiety, (b) depression, (c) substance abuse, (d) regression and dependency; and (e) denial.

Anxiety

Anxiety is common m plastic surgery patients. Some patients experience anxiety regarding anesthesia or worry that surgical reconstruction will not be completed. For some patients, anxiety is triggered by providing personal information or being physically examined, which are routine for the medical staff but stressful for many patients. Some patients fear loss of control and/or pain.

There are many forms of anxiety response, ranging in intensity from mild to severe. Surgeons should monitor patient symptoms of physiologic overarousal, worry, and generalized tension, and evaluate the degree to which these impact patient functioning (e.g .. sleep patterns).

One anxiety disorder of particular relevance to patients who have sustained traumatic injury is posttraumatic stress disorder (PTSD). The symptoms of PTSD include reexperiencing the trauma (e.g.. dreaming about or having flashbacks of the traumatic event). Patients report symptoms of increased arousal (e.g., sleep difficulties or unusual levels of irritability, anger, or tension). Some patients experience symptoms involving the "avoidance of stimuli associated with the trauma and the numbing of general responsiveness". Such patients avoid talking about the trauma, in addition to avoiding any stimuli associated with the trauma (e.g., avoiding automobiles if they were injured one). They may also report the "inability to recall an important aspect of the trauma". Posttraumatic stress disorder symptoms are common in individuals sustaining hand injury, burn injury and facial trauma. For some patients, onset of symptoms occurs long after the trauma (i.e., 6 months or more). For all patients experiencing PTSD symptoms, there is great personal suffering and a negative effect on rehabilitation. The surgeon can begin to relieve this suffering by identifying and labeling the symptoms and providing the appropriate intervention.

Interventions for Anxiety Responses

Much patient anxiety can be relieved through proper use of reassurance and information. "Knowing the patient's specific fears leads the physician to the appropriate therapeutic interventions. ... If the physician wrongly presumes to know why the patient is anxious without asking, then the patient is likely to feel misunderstood."

In some instances, even when reassurance and information directly address the patient's specific concern, it is still not enough to quell patients' anxieties. In these instances, benzodiazepines can be helpful for short-term relief of anxiety symptoms; however, great care should be taken in their use. They have potential for physical and psychologic dependence and can exacerbate PTSD symptoms. They also have a synergistic effect with alcohol, which some individuals use to reduce symptoms of tension and sleep difficulties. Any long term (i.e., greater than 2 weeks) prescription of anti-anxiety medication should be monitored by a psychiatrist because of the potential for coexisting psychiatric disorder (e.g., depression) requiring different forms of treatment.

Deciding to recommend psychiatric consultation is based on the patient's anxiety response. Is it beyond what would he considered "normal" (e.g., some worry/tension regarding anesthesia or the surgical outcome). This determination is often difficult to make.[156]

Anxiety is usually a symptom of psychiatric disorder when it remains umealistic or out of proportion despite the physician's clarification and reassurance. Other signs that anxiety requires psychiatric intervention are sustained disruption of sleep or gastrointestinal functions, marked autonomic hyperarousal (tachycardia, sweating), and panic attacks. Psychiatric consultation should always be requested when anxiety fails to respond to low doses of benzodiazepines, is accompanied by psychosis, or renders the patient unable to participate in their medical care.

Depression

Plastic surgeons regularly encounter individuals with clinical levels of depression.

It is essential to recognize symptoms of depression so that the patient can be referred for the effective treatments currently available. Failure to identify and treat symptoms of depression can result in unnecessary patient suffering and negatively affect patient rehabilitation. In the most serious in-stances, this failure can result in patient suicide.

The defining characteristics of depression include: depressed mood, loss of interest in usual activities, significant weight loss or gain (5% change), changes in sleep patterns, loss of energy, persistent fatigue, feelings of worthlessness, current thoughts of death (including suicidal thoughts and preoccupation with any death-related topic), increased agitation/restlessness, as well as inability to concentrate or make decisions. The patient may report these symptoms or they may be observed by the family, physician, or other members of the health care team.

It is important to specify that there is no one defining symptom of depression. Rather, depression is most accurately described as a syndrome involving changes in mood, thinking, and biologic functions (sleeping, eating, sex) that negatively affects the individuals daily functioning.

---

156 Altamura C. Paluello MO, Clinical and subclinical body dismorphic disorder, Eur Arch Psychiatry Clinic neuroscience, 2001.

The challenge in managing depression is distinguishing between "normal" depression (i.e., a reasonable emotional response to trauma or illness) and depression requiring treatment. Patients experiencing normal degrees of depression retain their abilities to communicate, make decisions, and participate in their own care when encouraged to do so.

Depression usually constitutes a psychiatric disorder when depressed mood, hopelessness, worthlessness, withdrawal and vegetative symptoms (e.g., insomnia, anorexia, fatigue) are present and out of proportion to the coexisting medical illness. Urgent psychiatric referral should always be obtained when the patient is thinking about suicide or has depression with psychotic symptoms. Psychiatric consultation should also be obtained if less serious depression fails to improve with the physician's support and reassurance, if antidepressant medication is needed, or if patients remain too depressed to participate in their own health care and rehabilitation.

It is recommended that plastic surgeons not conduct the psychopharmacologic treatment of depression; because of the any developments in medication management and the critical issues of differential diagnosis, this is best addressed by psychiatrist. However, it is essential that surgeons maintain a willingness to monitor the treatment so that the patients do not feel abandoned.

Zavisnost od alkohola

Plastic surgeons regularly encounter individuals with alcohol-related problems. Some reconstructive surgery patients, particularly those with a family history of substance abuse o depression, may use alcohol to "self-medicate" the negative feelings often associated with disfigurement and the stress of undergoing reconstructive surgery. Alcohol use also plays a role in placing some individuals at risk for sustaining injury, and can negatively impact rehabilitation. The critical features of alcohol dependence include the continued use of alcohol despite knowledge that social, psychologic or physical problems result from this use. Additional signs include the individual spending an inordinate amount of time engaging in alcohol use or neglecting to perform important social roles as a result of alcohol use. Individuals with alcohol problems may also manifest intolerance or withdrawal symptoms.[157]

---

157 Ibid.

Some clues that a patient may be having problems with alcohol include the smell of alcohol on a patient during consultation or a comment from a family member. If the surgeon is concerned that an alcohol problem may exist, it is the reason to be able to inquire by simply stating "I do not want to intrude on your life, but I am concerned and would like to be of help if I can. I am wondering if you are having any difficulties related to alcohol."

Four screening questions, defined as the CAGE questionnaire are very helpful in identifying individuals with an alcohol-related problem:

Cut down. Have you ever felt that you should cut down on your drinking?

Annoyed. Have other people annoyed you by criticizing your drinking?

Guilt. Have you ever felt guilty about drinking?

Eye-opener. Have you ever taken a drink in the morning to steady your nerves or to get rid of hangover?

If the patient answers yes to anyone of these questions, a more complete evaluation is warranted. However, the most difficult challenge in evaluating alcohol abuse is that patients, families, and physicians are prone in deny alcohol-related problems and choose to ignore signs and symptoms that are evident. It is not the surgeon's responsibility to ensure that patients obtain evaluation or treatment. However, it is the surgeon's responsibility to recognize and respond to signs that may be evident to review the above screening questions, and to present the availability of evaluation and treatment options in a compelling and compassionate manner.

Additional Psychiatric Problems

In addition to the psychologic responses already described, there are many others evident in reconstructive surgery patients. For example, some patients become extremely dependent and emotionally regressed when under pre- or postoperative stress. These patients behave in a childlike manner, often requiring massive amounts of support and reassurance. Other patients will evidence denial of their illness or disfigurement. Denial can be adaptive in some reconstructive surgery patients. If patient denial does not interfere with treatment, there is no reason to intervene.

However, when patient denial can lead to harm, then the surgeon needs to address it most likely by enlisting the help of both the family and a psychiatric consultant.

Other psychiatric problems encountered by plastic surgeons include delirium, dementia, substance withdrawal, and prolonged painÂmanagement problems. Additionally, patients may be suspected of malingering (i.e.. lying for the purposes of gaining money, workmen's compensation, or some other external gain) or factitious disorder (i.e., disorders that are self-created in order to take on the sick role). These disorders are all occasionally encountered by most plastic surgeons. Psychiatric referral is essential for each.

Factors Influencing Psychologic Adaptation to Disfigurement

Psychologic adaptation to disfigurement and surgical reconstruction is unique for each individual and is influenced by many factors including the etiology, salience and extent of the disfigurement as well as the individual's age and gender.

ETIOLOGY OF DISFIGUREMENT

Plastic surgeons generally need to provide more emotional support to patients with an acquired disfigurement than to patients with congenital disfigurement. Many psychologic challenges are inherent in adapting to congenital disfigurement. However, it is more psychologically disruptive to sustain a traumatic disfigurement than to have congenital disfigurement.

With congenital anomalies, there is time to incorporate the malformation into a sense of self. The individual may not like what is reflected in the mirror, but recognizes the image as his/her own, for better or worse. Further, there is a lifetime to prepare for the problems of being identifiably different. The trauma patient has had a lifetime of looking one way, and now must cope with looking both different and worse.

Changes in appearance, body image, and identity, along with stresses inherent in surgical treatment make it necessary that the surgeon spend extra time to ensure that patients with acquired disfigurement are understood and their concerns addressed. It is also more likely that they will present with acute symptoms of emotional disturbance (e.g anxiety, depression substance abuse) requiring psychiatric intervention.

SALIENCE AND EXTENT OF DISFIGUREMENT

There is no way to predict which patients will require increased psycho logic support on the basis of the salience or the extent of their disfigurement. It is well known that there is no necessary correlation between the extent of disfigurement and the degree of emotional response.

The consistent negative social response to facial disfigurement and the unique functional and aesthetic impact of hand injuries are massive challenges to psychologic adaptation. However, consistent with the subjectivity of body image responses, some individuals with a disfigurement hidden from view can be dramatically affected. For example, the impact of mastectomy and breast reconstruction is well documented, as are the problems with breast burns. However, the impact of "hidden injuries" is not necessarily limited to those areas of the body that are emotionally loaded (e.g., breasts and genitals).

DEVELOPMENTAL STAGE A D GENDER

A few generalizations can be made regarding developmental stage and psychologic adaptation to disfigurement. Disfigurement acquired before 2 years of age, and which does not progress over time, is more likely to result in psychologic adaptation similar to that of individuals with congenital deformities. School-age children and adolescents with a congenital or acquired disfigurement are more likely to experience increases in social and psychologic disruption.

Predictions regarding psychologic adaptation in relation to gender are very difficult to make. Females are subject to, and have internalized, more stringent standards regarding physical appearance, making it more likely that adapting to disfigurement will be difficult However, women are able to more readily adapt to body changes than are males. At present, no clear generalizations can he made, except that it is not safe to assume that adjustment to disfigurement is necessarily more difficult for women.[158]

---

158 Altamura C. Paluello MO, Clinical and subclinical body dismorphic disorder, Eur Arch Psychiatry Clinic neuroscience, 200 I.

SUMMARY

Many additional factors can influence patients' psychologic adaptation. Perhaps one of the most important is the degree of social support experienced by the patient. This support can come from family, friends, the community, the physician and ideally from many available sources. In general, patients with traumatic disfigurement who have little social support and poor pre-injury social and psychologic functioning are in greatest need of psychologic intervention.

Rehabilitation Interventions for Reconstructive Surgery Patients

Many reconstructive surgery patients who do not have identifiable psychiatric disturbances or profound negative psychologic reactions still experience the emotional challenges inherent in having any form of disfigurement. Much can be done to facilitate their rehabilitation, including making available the following resources: (a) networking and support groups, (b) techniques of image enhancement, (c) social skills interventions, and (d) body image therapy. Plastic surgeons play a pivotal role in ensuring that patients obtain those rehabilitation services.

NETWORKING AND SUPPORT GROUPS

Many patient support groups and networks are currently available and are valuable in providing patients with information and emotional support. For example, for those individuals with a facial disfigurement, there are numerous resources, which are often designed to serve specific populations (e.g., the Phoenix Society for bum survivors, and SPOHNC, a support group for people with oral and head and neck cancer). A helpful compilation of resources is available.

SOCIAL SKILLS TRAINING

Many individuals with facial disfigurement have difficulty in establishing positive patterns of interpersonal communication. These difficulties are largely due to the negative social reaction of those who are not disfigured. However, the patient's maladaptive patterns of coping may also contribute to this social strain. Whatever the source of social strain, the responsibility for improving patterns of interpersonal relations falls to the individual with disfigurement. Successful programs for teaching social skills to cope with disfigurement exist. One well-development program,

"Changing Faces", has been found to reduce social anxiety and improve self-confidence, and led to the development of the Disfigurement Recovery Unit at Frenchlay Hospital in Bristol, England. Similar services must be made accessible to all patients who desire to learn disfigurement related rehabilitation.[159]

IMAGE ENHANCEMENT

Image enhancement techniques, utilizing corrective cosmetics, personal grooming techniques, and development of effective nonverbal behavior exist for individuals with disfigurement. These techniques have been integrated into a well-developed program by Barbara Kammerer Quayle at the Center for Image Enhancement in cooperation with Department of Plastic Surgery at Ranchos Los Amigos Medical Center. The Image Enhancement Center provides interventions focusing on the use of corrective cosmetics, color analysis, color coordination, and the development of communication skills. Image enhancement facilitates the rehabilitation of individuals with facial disfigurement by providing effective techniques the individual can use to reduce the negative social response to their disfigurement and empowering the individual to take control over their own body image.

BODY IMAGE THERAPY

One set of techniques that has great potential for facilitating positive rehabilitation of individuals with any form of disfigurement is based on recently developed body image therapies. For individuals who habitually engage in negative and critical thinking about their appearance, who believe themselves to be unlovable as a result of their disfigurement, or who experience persistent and debilitating body image behaviors or notions, these interventions hold promise. Future plastic surgery rehabilitation programs will effectively employ these techniques to enhance the positive changes in appearance brought about by plastic surgery.

Conclusion

Plastic surgeons have the magnificent ability to improve patient appearance, body image, and overall psychologic motioning. By developing their abilities to understand and manage the psychologic dynamics of patients, surgeons can more effectively facilitate patient improvements in quality of life.

---

159 Ibid.

7. BASIC MEDICAL-LEGAL PRINCIPLES IN THE PRACTICE OF COSMETIC (PLASTIC) SURGERY

Medicine comprises the art of the prevention, palliation, and healing of illness. As early as 2000 B.C., the Code of Hammurabi documented concern for the quality of medical practice, which was once again emphasized in the Oath of Hippocrates in the 4th century, B.C. According to early English common law, a physician's liability was based on the fact that he was a member of a public calling, much like a shopkeeper.

The exchange of goods and services among individuals has resulted from society's existence. Such exchanges generate rights, obligations, and liabilities between the involved parties. With the rise of commercialism, the physician's role developed from a creation of contract law.

Torts principles and negligence law have supplanted contact law as the dictating doctrines of professional medical liability.

The moral and ethical responsibilities associated with the practice of medicine are well recognized, but the legal obligations between physician and patient are often less well understood. The current medical-legal climate would seem to dictate that the concepts of "duty," "negligence," "proximate cause" and "standard of care" should be included in the education of a surgeon just as are other principles of surgical management. This chapter will provide a brief overview of the legal obligations and risks inherent in the practice of medicine, with particular emphasis on plastic surgery. The information presented is generic and does not address jurisdictional differences. Since it is written by a surgeon and not in attorney, all statements are subject to legal review.

Physician-Patient Relationship

Certain characteristics of the physician-patient relationship make it distinctive. There is a basic difference between the individuals' knowledge bases; the patient carries with him a robe of frailty or vulnerability; the physician's sense of duty governs his actions, and it is hoped that a bond of trust exists.

A physician-patient relationship may be based upon a contract between parties (contractual *basis*), or on an undertaking to perform (*tort basis*), or on a combination of the two. For the purpose of personal injury cases, the consensual arrangement reached by the patient and physician "creates a status or relation rather than a contract".

Fault-Based Liability

For the most part, medical malpractice law is founded on a system of loss allocation that is based on the "fault" of the defendant. Liability without fault may be present in cases of *res ipsa loquitur,* lack of informed consent or breach of contract (e.g. in cases where guaranteed, specific results did not result). Nevertheless, usually some form of unacceptable conduct by the defendant or by someone for whom the defendant is responsible (*superior respondeat*) occurs.

In the majority of cases, the patient claims that the physician failed to perform according to the required standard of care. Regardless of the contractual or tort basis of the claim, the duty of care is usually the same.

Elements of a Negligence Claim

Legal actions pertaining to injuries coincident with the rendering of medical services are pursued as "personal injury claims." Three conditions[160] must be met if the legal definition of medical negligence is to be proven:

A series of events occur during the course of medical treatment.

A standard of care appropriate to these circumstances must be established.

The events that occurred during the course of medical treatment must then be proven to represent a significant departure from the established standard of care standard established by law for the protection of others against unreasonable risk of harm. In order to establish a valid negligence claim, the following elements must exist: (a) *a duty of care* was owed by the physician to the patient; (b) the physician violated the applicable *standard of care;* (c) the patient suffered *a compensable loss or injury;* and (d) such an injury was *caused in fact or proximately caused* by the substandard care. The burden of proving the existence of the above mentioned lies with the plaintiff (i.e., the patient or the patient's estate).

---

160 *Coleman v. California Friends* Chuck, 81 P 2d 469,470, Cal 1938; *Schneider v. Lillie Company,* I 5 I NW, 588, Mich 1915; *Pike v. Hon-singer,* 49 E 760, NY 1898; "The Standard of Care, Parts I, II, and III," 225 *JAMA* No. 6, page 671, August 3, 1973; 225 JAMA No. 7, page 791, August 13, 1973, 225 JAMA Mo. 8, page 1027, August 20, 1973; *Adkins v. Ropp,* 14 NE 2d 727, Ind 1938.

Duty

Contractual Creation of Duty

An expressed contract is created when a physician agrees to treat the patient in exchange for compensation; the courts will infer the presence of an implied contract where circumstances such as the institution of treatment with the patient's consent and with the expectation of compensation from the physician exist. The duty that is created is envisioned as being based on a service contract.

Once a physician-patient relationship is established, the duty of care demanded of a physician is imposed via the enforcement of tort law rather than as a result of any existing contract between the patient and physician. The exception to this premise arises when a special agreement has been created between the two parties, such as the guarantee of a specific result (e.g., the assurance that the surgeon can achieve the result visualized by the patient on a computer image). In the absence of such a special guarantee or agreement, the initial contract is important solely in the establishment of a professional relationship upon which the physician's duty is created.

Duty Created as a Result of Undertaking to Render Medical Care

A physician who undertakes to render care to a patient thus creates a professional relationship that carries with it a corresponding duty of care owed to the patient. According to this "undertaking" theory, the existence of the physician-patient relationship and its accompanying duty is not dependent upon payment for the physician's services.

Duty does not prevent the physician from refusing to prescribe treatment or refusing to perform a procedure which the physician does not believe is indicated,[161] but the physician cannot refuse to provide care once the professional relationship is established.

Duration of Duty

This duty remains in force until it is terminated in one of the three following ways:

---

161 Suburban Hospital Association v. Mewhinney, 187 A 2d 671, Md 1963.

137

By the patient's request. The patient may request that records and care be transferred to another physician, and from that point no longer receives care from the first physician.[162]

By mutual agreement. If there is no medical need for further services, the patient is informed and the relationship is terminated. Such termination usually requires no written communication to the patient, but an appropriate entry must be placed in the medical record. Referral or transfer of care to another physician with the patient's knowledge and consent can also terminate the relationship.

By the physician's request. A physician may end the relationship, but must meet more exacting requirements to insure continuity of care. The physician is not entitled to terminate the relationship unless reasonable advance notice is first given. The definition of reasonable advance notice depends on the patient's condition and the availability of other suitable care. The patient should be notified far enough in advance for the patient to acquire the effective management of another suitable physician. In order for the notice to be reasonable, it should apprise the patient of medical status and type of future medical care, including specialized care, needed.

Documentation is required, showing that the patient was duly notified (e.g. "As of 7 days from the receipt of this letter [or some other suitable time interval that conforms to local standards], I will no longer be responsible for your medical care"). The letter should be registered and a return receipt requested. An attorney acquainted with the requirements for terminating services to patients should be consulted regarding specifics that may apply to the surgeon's own region or jurisdiction.[163]

---

162 Miles v. Harris, 194 SW 839, Tex 1917.
163 Dashiell v. Griffith, 35 At! 1094, Md 1896; Capps v. Valk, 369 P2d 238, Kans 1962.

Abandonment

Unless the relationship is terminated by one of the alternatives listed above, the physician remains obligated to provide needed care to the patient. This obligation is without regard for any financial considerations. The inability or failure of the patient to pay for services rendered does not relieve the physician of the "duty" to continue to provide medical care.[164] Failure to respond to the medical needs of a patient because of unpaid bills may meet the legal definition of abandonment, a departure from the recognized standard of care; if damages occur, abandonment may result in a judgment against the physician.[165]

When the professional relationship between physician and patient is terminated unilaterally by the physician without reasonable notice or justification, or is unreasonably interrupted by a failure to treat the patient, the legal definition of abandonment has been met. For various professional or personal reasons, a physician may need to find a substitute physician to act in his absence. If, without justification, competent substitute physician is selected to care for the patient and harm proximally results as a result of the substitution, the physician may be liable if notice is not given in sufficient time for the patient to engage a physician of the patient's choice.[166]

If the physician prematurely terminates the patient's continuing need for care, the patient has been *intentionally abandoned* and the physician may also be liable for breach of contract. In such cases of conscious abandonment, the fact that the relationship was terminated may establish the physician's fault.

A patient's failure to return for follow-up care does not relieve the physician of the obligation to provide follow-up care. If such followup care is necessary to achieve a satisfactory result or maintain adequate control of a disease process, the physician has a responsibility to notify the patient of the need for continuing care.[167]

---

164 *McNevins v. Lowe*, 40 111 209, 111 1866; *Ritchey v. West*, 23 111 329, 111 1860; *Bomes v. Gardner*, 9 NYS 2d 785, NY 1939.
165 *Stohlman v. Davis*, 220 NW 247, Neb 1928; *Mucci v. Houghton*, 57 W 305, Iowa 1864; *Groce v. Myers*, 29 SE 2d 553, C 1944; McIntire, Leon L. The Action of Abandonment in Medical Malpractice Litigation. *Tulane Law Rev* 834, 1962.
166 *Miller v. Dore*, 154 Me. 363, 148 A.2d 692 (1959).
167 *Doan v. Griffith*, 402 SW 2d 855 Ky 1966; *Christy v. Saliterman*, 179 NW 2d 288, Minn 1970; *Welch v. Frisbie Memorial Hospital*, 9 A 2d 761, NH 1939.

Standard of Care: The Nature of the Duty Owed

Individuals must abide by certain standards of behavior in order to prevent avoidable injuries to others. If an injury occurs as a result of a deviation from these standards, the victim may bring action against the responsible party and may also be entitled to compensation.

Conduct is judged based on objective criteria. It is not sufficient that a physician perform to utmost potential and with utter good faith. Rather, the physician must conform to the standard of a reasonable person *under like circumstances.*[168] The standard that we as physicians are held to differs from that of the reasonable-person standard based on the following premises: (a) physicians are expected to possess and implement knowledge and skill in their professional practice that surpasses that of ordinary individuals; (b) the possession of such skill and knowledge has normally been evaluated as a result of professional standards set by the profession.

LEGAL DEFINITION

A physician is under a duty to use that degree of care and skill which is expected of a reasonably competent practitioner in the same class to which he belongs, acting in the same or similar circumstances.

Locality is merely one factor to be taken into account in applying general professional standards. The standard should be established by the medical profession itself and not by lay courts.

The evidence may include the elements of locality, availability of facilities, specialization or general practice, proximity of specialists and special facilities, as well as other relevant considerations.

---

168 Restatement 283.

PROFESSIONAL STANDARDS AND EXPERT TESTIMONY REQUIREMENT

The existence of a deviation from the standard of care must be proven as a result of expert testimony. The testimony of an "expert" is generally considered legally mandatory in medical negligence cases. Failure on the part of the plaintiff to provide expert testimony may result in a summary judgment in favor of the defendant physician without regard for any other circumstances in the claim. Only on very rare occasions is expert testimony not required. One example is that of *res ipsa loquitur* claim (it speaks for itself) in which acts of negligence are so obvious that courts have held that jurors can understand them without expert help.[169] Another example is the claim in which the physician openly admits liability and blame either at the time of the event or in subsequent testimony.[170]

Since specialists are examined by national certifying boards, specialists will generally be held to a national standard that permits testimony by experts from locales well outside the defendant's community.[171] Defendant physicians are held only to the standards of care that the average careful and prudent practitioner of their specialty would be expected to meet under the same circumstances.[172]

Whereas the events, or series of events, that occur in any given claim may be a matter of record, the standard or care appropriate to the circumstances can only be established through the testimony of a recognized "medical expert." The medical expert must not only testify as to the standard of care but also be willing to testify that the events of the claim represent a deviation from the established standard of care. It is not enough merely for the medical expert to testify as to what he would have done. The "medical expert" should possess the credentials and qualifications to establish the standard of care and, is usually, but not always, from the defendant's own specialty. Medical experts from other specialties may testify, but defendant physicians are usually held only to the standards that apply to their specialty or to their level of expertise.[173]

---

169 "Re Ipsa Loquitur, Parts I-VII" 221 *JAMA* No. 5, page 537, July 31, 1972; 221 JAMA No. 6, page 633, Aug 7, 1972; 221 *JAMA* No. I 0, page 120 I, Sept. 4, 1972; 221 JAMA No. 11, page 1329, Sept. 11, 1972; 221 JAMA o. 12, page 1441, Sept. 18,1972; 221 *JAMA* No. 13, page 1587, Sept. 25, 1972; 222 *JAMA* No. I, page 121, Oct. 2, 1972.
170 Holder AR. *Medical malpractice law.* New York: Wiley, 1975; 60.
171 *Hundley v. Martinez,* 158 SE 2d 159, W Va 1967.
172 "Standard of Care for Speciali ts Parts I and 11," 226 *JAMA* o. 2, page 251, October 8, 1973; 226 JAMA No. 3, page 395, October 15, 1973.

Time Frame of Reference

For the purposes of establishing negligence, a defendant's conduct will be evaluated in terms of the state of medical science and the professional standards as they existed at the time of the allegedly wrongful conduct.

Geographic Frame of Reference

The courts used to define the standard of care of the medical profession based on a reference to a limited geographical setting. This "strict locality rule" is now followed in only a small number of jurisdictions.[174] The rule is objectionable, based on the potential effect of maintaining small pockets of substandard practices in certain locales and on limiting the number of available expert witnesses.

"Respectable Minority" and "Error in Judgment"

In order to allow for differing viewpoints and opinions, the courts have developed a "respectable minority" rule. "A physician does not incur liability merely by electing to pursue one of several recognized courses of treatment."[175] Additionally, secondary to the fact that medicine is not an exact science, the "error in judgment" concept has been developed. This rule holds that a physician who otherwise follows the applicable professional standards should not be found liable merely because the decision turns out to have been the wrong one. This "error in judgment" rule does not determine the outcome of a case. Rather, this rule is given to the jury in their instructions. One court has observed, "errors in judgment which occur with the best intentions constitute negligence if they result from a failure to use reasonable care."

"Best Judgment" Rule

Some courts have held that it is not enough for a physician to comply with the professional standards of conduct. "If a physician fails to employ his expertise or best judgment, he should not automatically be freed from liability because in fact he adhered to acceptable practice. A physician should use his best judgment and whatever superior knowledge, skill and intelligence he has."[176]

---

174 Del.CodeAnn.18 6801 (&)Supp.1984).
175 *Downer v. Veilleux*, 322 A.2d 82, 87 (Me.1974); *Sprowl v. Ward*, 441 So.2d 898, 900 (Ala. 1983).
176 *Toth v. Comm. Hosp.* At Glen Cove, 22 N.Y.2d 255,263 & n 2,292 N.Y.S.2d 440, 447-448 & n. 2,239 N.E.2d 368,373 & n. 2 (1968).

Circumstantial Evidence and *Res Ipsa Loquitur*

Negligence may be proven in two different ways. It may be proven through the use of direct evidence, where the series of events that led to the injury and its accompanying negligence are explained. Additionally, negligence may be proven indirectly via circumstantial evidence. This indirect method of establishing negligence is referred to as the doctrine of *res ipsa loquitur,* "the thing speaks for itself."

Three elements must be present for the doctrine of res ipsa loquitur to apply. The insult must have:

resulted from an event that ordinarily doesn't occur in the absence of negligence.

been caused by an agency or instrumentality under the exclusive control or management of the defendant.

occurred under circumstances indicating that the injury was not due to any negligence or voluntary act on the part of the plaintiff.[177]

The most common factual pattern in which-the doctrine of *res ipsa loquitur* applies involves allegation of surgical sponges or instruments being left inside a patient. Additionally, courts have been more than willing to apply the doctrine to cases involving bums or trauma to parts of the patient's body not in the immediate operative field.[178]

Vicarious Liability

Besides being responsible for one's own actions, the physician may be legally responsible and held liable for the actions or omissions of others. For this doctrine of vicarious liability to be present, two conditions must be met:

A required relationship must exist between parties 1 and 2. This usually comprises that of an employer/employee relationship. Other relationships, such as "borrowed servants" relationships and partnership relationships, are also included.

---

177 *Loizzo v. St. Francis Hosp.,* 121 111.App. 3d 172, 76 III Dec 677,459 .E.2d 314,3 I 7 (1984).
178 Annot., 37 A.L.R.2d 464 (I 971, Supp. 1984).

The second requirement is that party 2 must have been acting within the contemplated scope of the relationship when the tort was committed. In an employer/employee relationship, the employee must have been acting within the "scope of his employment."

A physician may occasionally be held vicariously liable for the malpractice of another physician. These situations include those in which (a) one physician is the employee of another; (b) two or more physicians are partners or satisfy the requirements to be deemed members of a "joint enterprise"; and (c) when one physician is held to be a "borrowed servant" of another physician.[179]

"BORROWED SERVANT" RULE

The "borrowed servant" rule states: "A servant directed or permitted by his master to perform services for another may become the servant of such other in performing the services."[180] This theory applies to support staff such as residents, interns, nurses, and medical technicians, among others. The main question that has to be answered is whether a master/ servant relationship existed between the physician and the support staff despite the absence of a traditional employment relationship. Borrowed servant status depends upon a finding that the physician possessed the *required degree of control* over the staff person or resident.

In order to impose the threat of vicarious liability here, it must be shown that:

the support staff person was negligent.

the physician possessed the required degree of control over the staff support person.

the assistant was acting within the scope of his role as an assistant.

Direct negligence on the part of the physician need not be proven.

---

179 Franklin M, Rabin R. *Tort law and alternatives: cases and materials* 4th ed. New York: Foundation Press, 1987; 17.
180 The Restatement (Second) of Agency 227 (1958).

RESPONSIBILITY FOR OTHER PHYSICIANS

Many physicians may be involved in the performance of an operation besides the primary surgeon: anesthesiologists, residents, and interns, among others. The courts have been reluctant to characterize the participation of other specialists as that of borrowed servants. In the affirmation of the verdict for a surgeon, the court held that the surgeon could not be held vicariously liable for the actions of the anesthesiologist over whose performance she or he had (in the absence of evidence to the contrary) no control or right to control.[181]

RESPONDENT SUPERIOR THEORY

If one physician is employed by another, the supervising or employer physician can be held liable for the actions of the employed physician. If the physician is found to be an "independent contractor," the employer/employee relationship vanishes. Whenever there exists a formal relationship and involvement of wages and the right to control the manner of performance, as in a master/servant or employer/employee relationship, vicarious liability may be applied.[182]

PARTNERSHIPS AND PROFESSIONAL CORPORATIONS

A physician may be held vicariously liable for the torts of another physician who is a partnership member for conduct committed in the scope of partnership activities. Partners may also be held vicariously liable for the wrongdoings of the employees of the partnership.[183]

---

181 *Marvulli v. Elshire,* 27 Cal.App.3d 180. 103 Cal.Rptr. 461 (1972); *Accord Thompson v. Presbyterian Hosp., Inc.,* 652 P2d 260 (Okla. 1982)
182 Franklin M, Rabin R. *Tort law and alternatives: cases and materials* 4th ed. New York: Foundation Press, 1987; 17.
183 Crane J. Bromberg A. Bromberg, Law of Partner hip 64 (1968).

Causation Test

The time-honored test of causation is the "but for" or sine qua non test. Causation exists when the injury or loss would not have occurred "but for" the defendant's negligent conduct. An alternate test for causation has been that of the defendant's tortious conduct having been a "substantial factor" in bringing about the injury. Causation must be established by the standard of proof of a preponderance of the evidence. This requires the plaintiff prove that it was "more likely than not" that the defendant's negligence caused the harm.[184]

Proximate Cause

In addition to proof of negligence and proof of damages, the plaintiff is required to prove that the two are directly related, which is known as proximate cause.[185]

Damages

In addition to proving negligence, a claim for personal injury must establish proof of "damages." The plaintiff must show that damages have occurred that can be translated into monetary relief or retribution. The loss of income and/or the cost of care and treatment that results from a temporary or permanent disability due to negligence comprise economic losses. Claims for noneconomic losses such as "pain and suffering" may also be made. Proof of the existence of damages is essential to a medical liability claim. Even in the face of proven negligence, judgments have not been awarded unless damages occurred.[186]

JUDGMENT

When a claim of damages causally related to medical negligence is proven, the plaintiff will be entitled to a judgment that is usually monetary in nature and is satisfied through a transfer of assets from the defendant to the plaintiff. Unless there is some other source of compensation, such as medical liability insurance, the defendant's personal assets will be used to satisfy the judgment.

---

184 *Miles v. Edward O. Tabor, MD., Inc.,* 387 Mass. 783,443 .E.2d 1302 (1982); *Harvey v. Fridley Med. Center,* 315 .W.2d 225 (Minn. 1982).

185 "Proximate Cause, Parts I, II and III," *JAMA* No. 9, page 1479, Nov. 29 1971; 218 *JAMA* No. 10, page 1617, ec. 6, 1971; 218 *JAMA* No. LI page 1761, Dec. 13,1971.

186 *Morse v. Morelli,* 403 F 2d 564, CAOC 1968.

Medical Liability Insurance

To protect personal assets, physicians generally carry medical liability insurance. Premiums for such insurance vary widely according to risk, which is influenced by geography, specialty, and previous claims. Surgical specialties are rated by underwriters as possessing significantly higher risks than medical specialties. Plastic surgery is rated as a high-risk specialty because of the specialty's high frequency of claims, even though paid claims show relatively low average severity (i.e., size of award).[187]

In addition to providing compensation to the plaintiff, the insurance company also covers legal expenses coincident with the claim. Consequently, the insurance carrier generally reserves the right to choose the defense attorneys. Through its claims adjusters, the insurance company may also provide advice and attempt to influence decisions regarding the defense of a claim and/or settlement. The physician's rights with regard to settlement and defense strategy may vary between carriers. Therefore, each physician must be familiar with the limitations and restrictions of the individual policy.

A physician may wish to employ a private attorney independently to advise and assist in the defense. If the claim is for in amount that exceeds the physician's insurance coverage, a private attorney should be retained to defend that portion of the claim for which the insurance carrier is not liable.[188]

In acquiring and maintaining medical liability insurance, one should become knowledgeable regarding the types and !amounts of coverage available. The "basic" medical liability policy establishes limits of liability on the part of the carrier: a maximum amount that will be provided for "each event" of (i.e., claim) and a maximum amount that will be covered for "all events" for any given year in which the policy is in effect. These limits may be expressed as $100,000/$300,000 limits, or some similar combination. Most companies have maximum limits for the liability covered on the "basic" policy. When, in the physician's judgment, these limits are insufficient to meet exposure, the physician may wish to obtain additional insurance (known as an "umbrella" policy) that will provide coverage in excess of basic coverage. A basic policy must be in effect before an underwriter will provide an umbrella policy.

---

187 Sowka MP, ed. *Naic: Malpractice Claims; Final Compilation; Medical Malpractice Closed Claims;* 1975-1978. 350 Bishops Way, Brookfield WI: NAIC, 1980.
188 Alton WG Jr. *Malpractice: a trial lawyer's advice far physicians.* Boston: Little, Brown, 1977; 144.

TYPES OF COVERAGE

Coverage types vary between companies and can be influenced by the medical-legal climate in any given locality. "Occurrence" policies cover the physician for any occurrence (i.e., that occurs during the period of time that the policy was in effect, regardless as to when the claim is made). Occurrence policies are particularly desirable in cases in which the statute of limitations may be extensive, such as in the treatment of children, when claims may be filed even after adulthood for medical events that were allegedly mismanaged during childhood. Since the statute of limitations begins at the time of discovery of the alleged medical negligence, which may not be at the time of the actual procedure, occurrence policies are advantageous in that coverage for these events is maintained in perpetuity, even though the claim may be filed many years after the treatment rendered and even though the physician may not be currently insured by the original carrier.

"Claims made" policies provide coverage exclusively for claims that are filed during the period that the policy is in effect, and only if the incident occurred while the physician was continuously insured under the "claims made" policy. If the policy is dropped, the insurance carrier's liability is terminated. A claim filed at a later date on behalf of an event that occurred during the period that the "claims made" policy was in effect will not be covered. Retired physicians and/or physicians who change insurance companies will not be covered for claims that arise from previous events, even though they occurred during the time that the "claims made" policy was in effect. In such an event, the company may offer "prior acts" coverage or a "reporting endorsement" (commonly known as a "tail"), which provides insurance for claims that occur prior to or beyond the "claims made" coverage. The premium for such supplemental coverage is at the insurer's discretion and is based on their actuarial estimate of the potential continuing risk to which the physician may be exposed for events that occurred in the physician's past practice experience.

"Going Bare"

Some physicians believe that medical liability insurance may be an invitation for claims and think that plaintiffs will be less likely to pursue a claim against a physician who does not carry insurance. Individuals who do not carry medical liability insurance are "going bare". Physicians who go bare are encountering increasing difficulties in obtaining hospital staff privileges. The bylaws of many hospitals dictate that its staff personnel must carry a minimum level of medical liability insurance in order to be eligible for staff membership.

Irrevocable Trusts

Should a physician have the right to determine the measures that will be taken to provide compensation to a medically injured patient? Should a physician be forced to carry medical liability insurance if the physician has developed some other suitable compensation alternative? A willing physician may place personal assets at risk as long as the assets available are adequate to meet the potential damages. An alternative to carrying "basic" medical malpractice insurance that appears to meet these requirements is called an "irrevocable trust".[189]

Actions That May Affect Coverage

Medical liability policies must be examined carefully and exclusions from coverage duly noted. A physician may invalidate coverage if he or she fraudulently concealed actions that were related to (or were in any way responsible for) a medical negligence claim. Some carriers use very restrictive language within their policies that may void coverage in cases where physicians have altered medical records to avoid liability. Coverage may be voided if a physician fails to notify an insurance company of a claim or a potential claim. Medical-liability policies generally do not cover fraud, slander, libel, damages arising from unauthorized disclosures, or assault and battery.[190]

Insurance companies offer liability coverage on an annual basis and are under no obligation to provide a physician with insurance beyond the end of the termed policy period. Companies are free to set their own premiums, usually subject to review by state insurance commissioners. If these premiums are approved, the physician must be willing to pay the premium or lose coverage. The carrier is also free to determine the nature of coverage to be offered (e.g., "occurrence" vs. "claims made").

---

189 DeMere M. Comments of a doctor-lawyer on Chapter 54. In: Goldwyn RM, ed. *The unfavorable result in plastic surgery.* Boston: Little, Brown, 1984; 1122.
190 Holder AR. *Medical malpractice law.* New York: Wiley, 1975; 260.

The Patient's Right to Information and Self-Determination

REQUIREMENT OF CONSENT

The consent that a patient renders may be implied, and it may also be directly given. The physician must act in good faith in believing that the manifestation of consent accurately reflected the patient's true willingness to undergo the procedure. A consent may be invalidated when it is obtained by duress or misrepresentation concerning the nature or extent of the harm, or when the patient is acting under serious misapprehension of which the defendant is aware concerning such matters.[191]

The fact that a patient consents to an operative procedure by one physician does not ordinarily constitute consent to the performance by a substitute physician. The original physician may be found liable.[192] Additionally, the substitute physician may be found liable in the absence of a valid consent or emergency situation.[193] If a team of physicians are to be involved, this should be explained to the patient and appropriate consents obtained.

Implied Consent

Examination and treatment of patients require the patient's permission and consent. In many instances of medical practice, the consent is "implied"[194] and covers many minor procedures of which the patient is fully aware, such as injections, drawing blood, manual examinations, or any other of the various procedures that make up the daily practice of medicine. The fact that the patient permits these procedures to be done "implies" the patient's consent. Implied consent is present in instances in which immediate treatment is needed to save a life or preserve an individual's well-being. A surgical procedure can be performed without written consent (as in the treatment of a minor, or a patient who is mentally incapacitated) when a parent, spouse, or guardian is unavailable.

---

191 Restatement § 892A(2)(a), 892B.
192 *Perna v. Pirozzi,* 92 N. J. 446,457 A.2d 431 (1983).
193 *Guebard v. Jabaay,* 117 Ul.App.3d l, 72 Ill.Dec. 498, 452 N.E.2d 751 (1983) (dicta).
194 *Lardan v. Kansas City Gas Co.,* l OF 2d 2634, DC Kans 1926; *Caldwell v. Missouri State Life Insurance Co.,* 230 SW 566; Ark 1921; Cameron, to use of Cameron v. Eynon, 3 A 2d 423, PA 1939.

Additionally, implied consent is present m the treatment of individuals who are unable to give consent because of unconsciousness or other incapacitating mental or physical conditions. The validity of such implied consents are predicated upon proof that, had treatment been delayed, the patient's health and/or life would have been threatened and a rational, alert, and prudent adult patient would have consented to the procedure.[195]

Informed Consent

Patients contemplating elective procedures in which risks are known and alternative treatments are available must be provided information pertaining to these alternatives and risks as well as information describing the consequences, if any, of nontreatment.[196] The information must be provided so as to permit the risks to be seen in proper perspective and to accurately transmit realistic expectations of the results of treatment.[197] The patient must then provide his/her personal consent for the procedure or treatment. Such consent is regarded as "informed" consent and is documented in written form, in which the patient acknowledges that this information was provided and that permission has been granted to perform the procedure. Informed consent is not static but is a continuing process in the patient's treatment, during which updated information must be regularly provided and the original content of the consultation continually reviewed.

Informed consent is never to be construed to be the consent form. No matter how complete or detailed the form, if the information therein has not been clearly transmitted to the patient, the patient is not "informed." Elaborate and lengthy consent forms may be appropriate for some regions and some practices. Short, simple forms written in understandable language with a section in which the patient has written in his/her own hand that they have received the information and have understood it may be equally effective or more so, in a court of law. The nature of the information provided to the patient must be fully documented in the patient's record.

---

195 Prosser WL. *The law of torts.* 4th ed. St. Paul, MN: West, 1971.
196 *Truman v. Thomas*, 661 P 2d 902, Cal 1980.
197 *Milchell v. Robinson*, 334 SW 2d 11, Mo 1960.

Informing The Patient

In order for the patient to be properly informed, the following information must be provided:

Nature of the disease, injury or deformity

Purposes and goals of treatment and consequences of nontreatment

Limitations of treatment and consequences of nontreatment.

Treatment alternative

Risks and complications of treatment

All information modalities should be contemplated as a means to inform and educate patients. While some patients may understand and retain information transmitted verbally, others will be more completely informed by providing additional written material, diagrams, and other appropriate audiovisual presentations. A notation as to the nature of the printed information or visual presentation that was provided should be made in the patient's record. In addition, copies of this supplementary material should be on file to document the information provided, should a question ever arise as to the nature of the information given.

Informed consent or the lack thereof does not possess the pivotal importance to plaintiff attorneys that surgeons often believe. Plaintiff attorneys focus on negligence, causation and damages. Failure to provide adequate information upon which a patient can make an "informed decision" may reflect an unacceptable standard of care,[198] but without the presence of damages, the sole lack of informed consent is not considered by most plaintiff attorneys to be an appropriate basis for a claim. However, in claims in which significant damage has occurred as a result of possible negligence, the lack of adequate "informed consent" can significantly reinforce the plaintiff's claim of negligence.

---

198 *Truman v. Thomas,* 661 P 2d 902, Cal 1980.

Some physicians believe that, having informed the patient of the potential for a complication, the patient has no basis for a claim if that complication occurs. No matter how thorough the consultation or how complete the list of complications, the physician does not invoke a claim of immunity for a complication if it occurred as a result of negligence.[199] When the patient has been adequately informed, she or he may be more likely to regard and more ready to accept complication as a known risk regardless of cause; but, if the complication is unexpected, a claim is more likely to occur, even if it can later be proven that the complication was a recognized and accepted risk of the surgical procedure and was not due to negligence.

Despite detailed efforts to inform, patients retain very little of the information provided. Excellent studies have shown that, in a matter of only a few days, the majority of information provided to patients cannot be recalled.[200] Even though some patients do not retain the information provided, efforts to inform the patient as completely as possible may be accompanied by a perception on the part of the patient that the physician is concerned, sensitive, and thorough. Transforming the uncertainties and fear of treatment into manageable realities, in which the patient and physician develop an alliance of mutual trust and understanding, may be a major factor in presenting negative reactions to treatment and prove to be a better claim deterrent than a legalistic lists of complications.[201]

The basic information upon which informed consent is given must be provided by the physician. The information provided by the physician can then be supplemented by associates, residents, nurses, or other qualified individuals, and can be further supplemented by printed material and/or audiovisual presentations.

---

199 *Mull v. Emory University,* 150 SE 2d 276, Ga I 966; Block.v. Mc Vay, 126 W 2d 808, SD I 964.

200 Gray BH. An assessment of institutional review committees in human experimentation. *Med Care* 1975; 8:318-328; Golden JS, Johnston GD. Problems of distortion in doctor-patient communications, *Psychiary and Medicine* 1970; 50:127-148; Lee D, Bowers DG, Lynch JB. Observations on the myth of "infonned consent." Plast Reconstr Surg 1976; 58:280-282.

201 Gutheil TG, Havens LL. The therapeutic alliance: contemporary meanings and confusions. *Int Rev Psychoanal* 1979; 6:467-681.

Validity of Consent

In a landmark decision upholding the right of patients to self-determination, Justice Cardozo wrote, "Every human being of adult years and sound mind has a right to determine what shall be done with his own body..." Strictly interpreted, valid consent for treatment can only be obtained from the patient. Special circumstances or "exceptions"[202] occur when patients are deemed incapable of participating in the consent process. These exceptions include minors, for whom consent must be obtained from a parent; patients who have been adjudicated by a court of law to be incompetent or incapable and for whom a consent must be obtained from the court-appointed guardian; and victims of emergencies, in which delays in treatment could result in a threat to the patient's medical well-being.

The existence of an emergency is determined by a physician and is a matter of medical judgment. Medical judgment, however, is subject to judicial review, and the physician's decision may be overruled. Invoking the emergency exception to obtaining consent should be reserved only for circumstances in which it is impractical to secure consent and when further delay would pose a significant risk to the patient. In situations in which patients cannot participate in decision making, a physician should, as current law requires, attempt to secure a relative's consent if possible, which is known as a "substitute consent". In the event that no one is available to provide a substitute consent, or when time does not permit locating an appropriate individual, the physician should carefully document the situation that precluded such efforts. Unsuccessful attempts to contact relatives should also be noted. In the absence of consent, it is prudent to obtain and document the opinion of a second physician regarding the necessity of emergency treatment, as long as this second opinion does not result in a delay harmful to the patient.

---

202 Meisel A. The "exceptions" to the infonned consent doctrine: striking a balance between competing values in medical deci ion making. *Wisconsin Law Review* 1979; 2:413-488.

When attempting to obtain a substitute consent, or when advising a family of a patient's condition, the physician must be sensitive to the confidentiality inherent in the doctor-patient relationship. The physician must guard against the disclosure of unnecessary details, facts, or information pertaining to the patient's medical condition to members of the family or "friends" that might later be found to be detrimental to the patient. Disclosures made to anyone without the patient's consent, even in cases of emergency, and even in cases where the information provided was for purposes of obtaining substitute consent, may later be the basis for a claim of "unauthorized disclosure" which, if accompanied by proven damages, could result in a judgment against the physician.

Consents should be written in language that can be understood by the average lay person.[203] Studies have shown that, to be effective, consent forms should be worded at no higher that the 7th or 8th grade level.[204] consent forms should be worded at no higher that the 7th or 8th grade level (53). Consent forms that list only the technical or medical terminology for a procedure may later be mischaracterized. A plaintiffs attorney may convince a jury that the language used in the form represents the terminology that was used during the consultation (i.e., that it was so technical and so thick with medical terms that no patient could understand what was being said). A thorough consultation provided in language that is easily understood by the average lay person should not be negated by a written consent that contains terms which can only be deciphered by a physician.

Consents must be obtained at a time when the patient is mentally capable of giving consent. Obtaining consent after the patient has received medication that could have altered the patient's mental capacity will invalidate the consent. Where patients appear mentally confused or mentally incompetent but have not been adjudicated incompetent, consent should still be obtained from the patient. Good medical practice would dictate that a responsible family member also be provided with as much information as is necessary to establish "informed consent". A signed statement from

---

203 *Pedesky v. Bleiberg,* 59 Cal Rptr 294, Cal 1967.
204 Gmnder TM. On the readability of surgical consent forms. *New Eng J Med* 1980; 302:896. Mohammed MB. Patients' understanding of written health infonnation. *Nurs Reg* 1964; 12: 100.

the family member to that effect should also be placed in the patient's record. To bypass the "confused patient" and accept consent only from a member of the family may later be complicated by a patient who has regained their senses and brings action not only for a medical misadventure but also for battery resulting from a lack of a valid consent.[205][206]

Having obtained consent for treatment, the physician is now obligated to manage the patient within the constraints of the consent provided. A surgeon may extend a procedure beyond that to which the patient agreed, but only if it can be shown that to do otherwise would have jeopardized the patient's medical well-being.[207]

The Importance of Medical Records

MEDICAL-LEGAL SIGNIFICANCE

The focus of all medical negligence claims is the medical record. The first documented information that is reviewed by the plaintiffs attorney is the medical record. An attorney's decision to accept or reject the case is usually based on the content and character of the medical record. If a suit is tried, the result for or against the defendant physician will be decided largely on the basis of the medical record. The importance of well-documented, timely, and complete medical records cannot be overemphasized in the defense of medical negligence claims and in its effectiveness in discouraging claims that might otherwise be filed a medical record is exactly what the name implies - a record of medical events. The purpose of the medical record is not to provide a defense in a legal action but to facilitate patient care and provide a record of that care. Some defense attorneys have suggested that the record should be written as though it were being read by a jury. Many physicians would disagree. Medical records should be written so as to provide pertinent information to physicians, nurses, technicians, and other health care providers to assist in the coordination of the patient's care. The record should be written so that, if the treating physician were suddenly incapacitated, another physician who previously knew nothing about the patient could immediately take over the patient's care with no interruption in the continuity of that care. A good medical record will, by definition, be a good legal record.

---

205 *Scholoendorff v. Society of New York Hospital,* 195 NE 92, NY 1914.
206 *Pedesky v. Bleiberg,* 59 Cal Rptr 294, Cal 1967.
207 *Kennedy v. Porrott,* 90 SE 2d 754, NC 1956; *Russell v. Jackson,* 221 P 2d 516, Wash 1950.

In the course of, a medical practice, a physician deals with hundreds of medical problems, many of them having great similarity. When one of the medical problems generates a claim of medical negligence, it is often difficult for the physician to recall from memory specifics relating to the claim. On the other hand, the patient who has filed the suit has probably only dealt with one medical problem that involves the defendant physician. Recollection of the event specifics and details are much more sharply focused in the patient's mind than they could ever be in the mind of the treating physician. It would seem that the patient and the patient's attorney would have a significant advantage. However, that advantage is usually neutralized by the fact that physicians keep contemporaneous written records and patients do not. An accurate, timely, well-documented medical record will always be regarded as carrying greater credibility in the eyes of an attorney and jury than the patient's undocumented recollections of events, most of which occurred months or years previously.

ACCURACY

As medical events occur in the treatment of a patient, words should be carefully chosen that transmit appropriate intent. Words like "inadvertent" to physicians may reflect harmless and unintentional acts, whereas the legal world sees inadvertance as negligence. The physician should be thorough in describing a condition, finding, or situation, but only to the point that it meets the needs of another physician. Long, defensive notes appearing in a record will only alert a perceptive attorney to an unusual occurrence that might otherwise remain insignificant.

Dictated, transcribed, and typewritten reports generate some of the most significant entries in a patient's record. This is a commonly accepted practice throughout hospitals and physicians' offices. Many of these lengthy reports are read very superficially or not at all before being signed by the physician. The signing of a record without an accompanying disclaimer indicates that the physician believes the report is a true and accurate record. In actual practice, transcription errors, typographical errors, inaudible words, unintentional omissions, and the incorrect choice of words to describe a clinical situation occur so frequently that careful line-by-line, word-by-word review of each dictated record should, theoretically, be mandatory before the physician applies a signature. Frequently, physicians fail to do so, and sign incomplete records or records that contain significant inaccuracies with no apparent effort to correct or complete the record. Attorneys may interpret such records as conveying indifference and inattention to detail on the part of the physician, which might further reinforce the attorney's impression that the physician may have also been indifferent and negligent in the medical treatment of their client.

Inaccuracies contained in records must be corrected contemporaneously. A single line should be drawn through an inaccurate entry and accompanied by the written correction, date, and physician's initials. It is absolutely essential that, in making a correction, the physician or other health care provider not erase, obliterate, or destroy any portion of the medical record. The words through which the line is drawn must still be legible.[208]

Numerous corrections, even though conforming to acceptable standards, that occur following the date that a suit was filed should be avoided. Before undertaking any corrections in a record that is subject to a lawsuit, the defendant physician should consult with the defense attorney as to recommendations regarding inaccurate entries that are present in the medical records.

TIMELINESS

Failure to dictate or write reports immediately may result in significant medical-legal problems for the defendant physician, should the record ever be part of a negligence claim. Records and reports that are dictated days to weeks (or more) after the medical event occurred will be discredited in a court of law. A plaintiffs attorney will convey to the jury that delinquent entries are either:

After the fact delinquent incident or circumstance descriptions that would satisfactorily explain an injury or complication, and which ordinarily would have no negligence attached, will be characterized as having been made after the surgeon was aware of the injury, and made purposely after the fact so as to diminish liability. Even though circumstances and all events within a delinquently dictated record may be accurate, and truly reflect the circumstances of the procedure, a question of doubt will be raised as to the validity of these entries because of the timing of the dictation.

---

208 Alton WG Jr. *Malpractice: a trial lawyer's advice for physicians.* Boston: Little, Brown, 1977; 81.

Not subject to accurate recall. A plaintiff's attorney can demonstrate a surgeon's inability accurately to recall events days or weeks later by asking the surgeon to provide details of other events of that particular day (that may have had nothing to do with the medical practice but that may appear to a jury to be events that should be remembered). Once the physician's failure accurately to recall events of the day is established, the jury is then led to believe that the precise events of the surgery could not be accurately remembered either.

Injuries that are largely due to contributory negligence on the part of the patient because of failure to follow instructions following discharge can later be construed by the plaintiff's attorney to be due to inadequate or incomplete discharge instructions on the part of the physician. If instructions appear only on a discharge summary that is dictated days to weeks after the physician would have been aware that the patient had failed to follow instructions, the discharge instructions appearing in the discharge summary will be discredited, even though it may be a true and accurate reflection of the instructions provided.

Legibility

For a medical record to perform the function for which it was intended, the entries must be legible and easily interpreted by other health care providers participating in the patient's care. Some physicians take perverse pride in the fact that their handwriting is illegible. Some believe that there is security in illegible handwriting because it can only be interpreted by the writer. However, illegible entries give an opposing attorney an opportunity to raise questions about every illegible entry and imply to the jury that these illegible entries actually say something other than what the physician is claiming or that the defendant physician is interpreting these entries to meet the physician's particular needs under the circumstances of the suit. Such inferences provide an opportunity for the plaintiffs attorney to suggest to a jury that the defendant physician may not be honest. This can be even more detrimental to a physician's defense than a demonstration of negligence.

Never obliterate an entry in the medical record. Any entry that has been rendered illegible provides the opposing attorney an opportunity to suggest to the jury that the obliterated entry contained the exact information that would have proven the defendant physician's negligence beyond a doubt when, in fact, the information obliterated may have been of rather minor significance. Nothing that the defendant physician may thereafter relate to the jury as having been contained in the obliterated entry will change the perception within the jury's mind that the obliterated entry was much more damaging.

VALIDITY

The jury must believe that the record is a true and accurate representation of the circumstances that occurred contemporaneous with the treatment. Accepted methods to correct inaccuracies within a record were described earlier in this chapter. Additions, deletions, or alterations of any kind made to a record without proper notation may, if proven, void a physician's malpractice insurance coverage and will frequently result in a verdict against the physician. Technology is currently available that can determine the point in time in which entries have been made as well as decipher entries which have been altered or rendered illegible to the naked eye. Medical records that have been found to have been altered without proper notation may attract a plaintiff's attorney, even though the case has no significant merit. If an altered record is proven to exist *the whole focus of the claim may be shifted from the alleged act of negligence to the question of the honesty and integrity of the physician.* If it can be shown that a physician has altered a record in an effort to avoid liability, juries will consider the physician dishonest. Plaintiffs attorneys are very aware that juries do not accept dishonesty in physicians and in such instances frequently choose to punish the physician with awards to the plaintiff which may actually have very little to do with the alleged act of negligence. An incomplete record or one with numerous inaccuracies can be defended much more easily than a record that has been surreptitiously altered.

Keeping the Patient Out of the Attorney's Office

Greater socioemotional overtones are present in medical-legal claims than in other personal injury claims. Some lawsuits suits may be triggered by events that have nothing to do with technical errors or negligence. In many cases the patient's first visit to the attorney's office may be prompted by an by emotional reaction to what the patient believes to be mistreatment, rather than any definite awareness of a medical mistake.

Anger in response to perceived indifference, lack of concern, sympathy, or attention is often the precipitating emotion that causes a patient to first seek legal advice. A plaintiff's attorney welcomes angry clients and wishes to learn what the physician did to make the patient angry. The circumstances can eventually be transmitted to a jury in hopes of making the jury angry as well.

When a patient consults an attorney, the attorney then has the opportunity to search the medical record for a basis for suit. The attorney may find a basis that otherwise may never have been discovered and, ironically, may be completely unrelated to the patient's reason for seeking legal advice. If the patient is sufficiently angry with the physician, the patient may accept any basis for a claim as a means of punishing the physician for the physician's "wrongdoing". **The single most effective way to prevent malpractice claims is to keep the patient out of the attorney's office.**

Factors that Cause Patients to Consult an Attorney

In addition to anger, financial hardship generated by injury, disease, surgery, complications, or financial pressure from a physician or hospital for payment of delinquent bills, especially following an unfavorable result, can result in a lawsuit. The patient may not be aware of any specific acts of medical negligence. Financial pressure may prompt the patient to seek legal advice in hopes of uncovering medical negligence that might serve as a basis for obtaining financial relief.

"Surprise" occurring as a result of an unexpected complication may cause patients to seek legal advice. Even though the complication may later be shown to have occurred without any negligence on the physician's part, the unexpected nature of the complication may cause the patient to believe otherwise. Such events can frequently be prevented through greater emphasis on the informing process, covered earlier in this chapter. Information provided before surgery will be regarded by the patient as "informed consent"; the exact same information provided after surgery will be regarded as "excuses".

Disappointment can also prompt a patient to consult an attorney if expectations from treatment remain unmet. If the expectations were unrealistic, or if the physician provided overly optimistic assurances, the fault may lie with the physician's inability to communicate. Failure to meet expectations may not be a basis for a claim of negligence, but the disappointment resulting from such a failure may cause the patient to consult an attorney, thereby permitting the attorney to review the record and possibly uncover an act of medical negligence that might have otherwise remained unformulated.

IDENTIFYING THE PATIENT POSSIBLY PLANNING TO SEEK LEGAL ADVICE

Expressions of personal dissatisfaction by a patient are the most direct evidence of a patient who may eventually seek legal advice. Other patients may demonstrate more subtle signs of dissatisfaction. Expressions of distress over a complication out of proportion to the event, or persistent focus on unmet expectations and an unwillingness to accept that "nothing more can be done" may be characteristics of patients who are likely to consult an attorney.

A dissatisfied patient who fails to return for follow-up care is frequently a patient who has sought medical attention elsewhere and/or plans to consult an attorney.

A litigious patient may display resentment over the need for additional surgery to correct a complication especially, if additional costs will occur. Such a patient may demonstrate inability to understand how a complication could occur without "something having gone wrong". Hostile statements made to the office or hospital staff, or to other patients, should alert the physician and staff to a patient who may be considering legal action. Patients are inclined to express dissatisfaction to others before expressing it to the physician. The staff should be aware of this and convey any information that will assist the physician in the reduction or modification of legal exposure.

Anger or frustration over a bill, billing techniques, or the handling of insurance claims may precede a visit to an attorney's office. The patient will almost certainly seek legal advice following an unfavorable result if pressure is applied for payment of the bill or if the bill is turned over to a collection agency. Hospitals are particularly prone to push for the collection of delinquent accounts even in cases in which patient dissatisfaction can be shown to be due to hospital-based negligence. Hospital-directed claims will almost always name the treating physician and therein involve the physician in a claim mat might possibly have been avoided through a more temperate management of hospital accounts. Physicians must personally monitor the handling of accounts of dissatisfied patients or patients with unfavorable results. This may include making inquiries of hospital billing departments as to the status of the patient's hospital account. Hospital administrators must be informed of dissatisfied patients or patients with unfavorable results to permit judgments to be made as to how the account should be managed, depending in part on the medical-legal implications of the event.

Dissatisfied patients who begin to appear for visits accompanied by relatives or friends (when previously the patient came to the office alone) may represent individuals who need the support of others to reinforce their contention that mistreatment has occurred and that consulting an attorney is justified.

Any inferences made to a physician suggesting that the patient may be considering legal action against some other medical provider should alert the physician and staff to the potential for being involved, even though the patient may make assurances to the contrary. All assurances may be negated once an attorney has an opportunity to review the case. Particularly difficult problems occur if one provider has supported the patient's contention that another provider may have been negligent, especially if such support was provided in hopes of deflecting liability.

MANAGING THE PATIENT POSSIBLY PLANNING TO SEEK LEGAL ADVICE

The physician must not wait for the patient to generate enough courage to express dissatisfaction. The physician may already be aware of dissatisfaction through information gleaned from others, or as demonstrated through information gleaned from others, or as demonstrated through behavior patterns outlined above. Early and direct intervention on the part of the physician in exposing the problem, and shared decision-making in its resolution, provide several advantages to the physician:

The physician is permitted to take the initiative by having already prepared recommendations and a plan of management to address the problem. This is preferable to having to develop them "on the spur of the moment" in a confrontational situation generated by the patient.

Time is minimized for the patient to "dwell" on the problem or exaggerating the problem.

The patient is deprived of the m1t1at1ve, thereby minimizing the patient's opportunity to develop an organized complaint.

Dissatisfied patients sometimes find it easier to express their concerns and disappointments in writing. Such letters deserve immediate attention. Writing letters in response to patient dissatisfaction is sometimes a more effective method of reacting than telephone calls or face-to-face confrontation, which can be intimidating to some patients. A letter gives the patient tangible evidence of the physician's concern. A letter can also be used by the patient to refute the contentions of the family members or friends or that the physician is indifferent or uncaring. The letter should be structured so as to express concern and sensitivity, but lengthy explanations or excuses should be avoided. The patient should be invited to return to the office and discuss the problem with the physician personally. Dissatisfied patients should also be urged to obtain a second opinion. If the patient is willing, such arrangements can be made by the treating physician, but the appearance of one physician "covering" for the other should be avoided. Patients may wish to make their own arrangements; in any case, the treating physician should offer to send a medical summary with the patient.

SEEING ANOTHER PHYSICIAN'S DISSATISFIED PATIENT

Second opinions are often sought by patients with unfavorable results. Seeing another physician's dissatisfied patient is one of the most difficult challenges that a physician will encounter in medical practice. Skillful management may diffuse a potential lawsuit. Conversely, lawsuits that might otherwise have been avoided have been filed because of remarks made by a consultant that were later found to be based on incomplete information and unwarranted assumptions.

When a physician sees another physician's dissatisfied patient for the first time, the consultant must exercise caution in, accepting the patient's account of the events of treatment until such time that records can be obtained from the treating physician. The patient's authorization must be provided before the consultant can obtain information regarding previous treatment. Contacting the treating physician without patient authorization could be regarded as a violation of confidentiality.

Frequently, patients do not wish to identify the treating physician. The consultant would be well-advised to inform the patient that proper evaluation of the patient's condition is not possible without obtaining previous records of treatment and without discussing the matter with the original physician. Consultants must be very cautious in accepting patients who persist in not wanting to identify the treating physician or not wanting the treating physician contacted. Such restraints can be used to justify withdrawing from case (i.e., "While I respect your request for confidentiality, I cannot properly evaluate your case without obtaining information from your original physician.").

During the course of evaluating the patient's condition, the consultant must avoid conveying by attitude, expression, or word that the condition is due to negligence on the part of the treating physician. To do so will establish this perception permanently in the minds of the patient and family. Nothing that may occur thereafter will change this perception. The patient now has a reason to consult an attorney, who will be advised that the treating physician is at fault because the consultant said so. If subsequent review of the patient's records indicates that the treating physician did not deviate from the standard of care and the consultant thereafter testifies to the same, both physicians will appear collusive in the eyes of the patient-the treating physician for having been negligent and the consultant for "covering up".

Consultants who examine dissatisfied patients must concentrate on an objective evaluation of the patient's *current* medical condition and avoid discussions of liability and fault. The patient must be made to understand that the consultant's function is to provide assistance to both the patient and the treating physician for the purpose of modifying the unfavorable result. Efforts by the consultant to influence the patient to focus on a positive remedial treatment plan rather than liability or fault will be in the best interest of all parties.

If the interests of the patient and treating physician would best be served by the patient's returning to the original physician, the consultant must do everything reasonable to encourage this. If the patient does not wish to return to the original physician, the consultant is not obligated to accept the patient. However, if the consultant does accept the patient, he or he will no longer be considered a consultant but rather a treating physician.

Patients who concentrate on placing blame for an unsatisfactory result and seem uninterested in any corrective treatment may have already consulted with an attorney. A patient may seek a consultation on the advice of his attorney and may not indicate the referral source. Unfortunately, once the patient has been seen, the consultant cannot avoid involvement in the lawsuit if one is filed.

INTENSIVE CARE FILE

Some patients are greater medical-legal risks than others and deserve closer monitoring. Establishing an intensive care file may be an effective method to monitor such patients.

To establish such a file, the physician must identify patients with unfavorable results, patients with complications, "dissatisfied" patients, and any other patient who appears to represent a particular medical-legal risk. These patients' charts or names can then be segregated into a special file of which each member of the physician's staff is aware. A strict policy must then be developed by which these patients are monitored at set intervals by the physician or a specifically designated member of the staff in regard to:

Current status

Date last seen

Adequacy and completeness of records

Security of records (protection from fire and theft)

Need for second opinion

Attitudes/reactions, both of patient and patient's family

All telephone conversations-written records

Any special preparation needed for the next office visit

Need for continued "intensive care" vs return to regular files.

POLICY MANUAL

Misunderstandings, communication errors, and inconsistencies in patient management by the office staff can sometimes generate, or further aggravate, patient dissatisfaction following an unfavorable result. Uniform policies governing the management of records, billing, telephone calls, appointments, and general communication guidelines should be developed by the physician and placed in a policy manual, which may then serve as an effective risk management tool in some practices. Such a manual must be "required reading" for the staff, and may be useful in introducing and teaching risk management concepts and techniques to the staff.

MAIL-0-GRAMS

Using Mail-O-Grams rather than registered letters may be preferable when contacting patients regarding problems with significant medical-legal overtones (e.g., the failure to return for follow-up care). A MailO-Gram does not carry the medical-legal stigma of a registered letter and yet projects urgency. A copy of the Mail-O-Gram, which can be placed in the patient's records, is provided to the sender.

PATIENT QUESTIONNAIRE

Confidential patient questionnaires serve not only as an effective risk management device but also as an effective practice development tool. What counts is what the patient thinks - not what the physician, colleagues, or staff think. The questionnaire must be made absolutely confidential and anonymous for "physician's eyes only" by mailing all responses to a P.O. box or to the physician's home. The following suggestions[209] can be varied or supplemented to suit one's own practice:

Communication. Do patients understand the diagnosis and the course of treatment being proposed? Do they understand what they are supposed to do after leaving the office? Do they feel they have not been told enough, talked down to, or not shown enough respect?

Professional services. Is the physician thorough enough? Does the physician spend enough time with the patient?

Office. Does the patient like the setting? Is the office up to date? Is it too crowded? Uncomfortable? Not private enough?

Staff. Are they courteous? Helpful? Knowledgeable? Confidential, and considerate of privacy? Available?

Practice. Are services readily available? Do patients have to wait too long to be seen? Do patients wait too long in the waiting room? Are billing and insurance procedures handled satisfactorily?

Does the patient have any other questions?

---

209 *Malpractice Digest.* St. Paul Fire and Marine Insurance Co. October 1984; 3.

Limitations on Liability and Defenses

STATUTE OF LIMITATIONS

Instances of alleged medical negligence must be acted upon by the plaintiff within a defined period of time following the act of negligence or the discovery of the act of negligence. In most cases, failure to institute legal action within this statutory period of time precludes a person from filing a lawsuit. In many jurisdictions, discovery rules[210] are applied to prevent the statute of limitations from precluding the filing of a suit in a situation where the patient would not have known the injury had occurred. In such instances, the statute of limitations begins only at the time that the alleged act of negligence was discovered by the patient, rather than being related to the time that the actual incident occurred.

Unfavorable results related to possible medical negligence must be disclosed to the patient, and the exact date and time that the disclosures were made must be documented in the medical record. The statute of limitations does not begin until the disclosure is made. Any intention to conceal such facts will prevent the statute of limitations from applying until such time that the disclosure is made. In addition, efforts to conceal an injury due to medical negligence may be regarded by the courts as "fraudulent concealment," which could affect medical-liability insurance coverage.

Statutes of limitations in most jurisdictions are shorter for personal-injury claims than statutes covering contract law. Physicians must avoid any statement or any written record that would suggest the patient has been given a "guarantee" in regard to the results of a surgical procedure or medical treatment. Such "guarantees" may be regarded by the courts as contractual agreements and, therefore, subject to the much longer statute of limitations for contracts rather than the shorter statutes for personal injury. Any diagrams, drawings, overlays, computer images, or plans of treatment based on cephalometrics, for example, should have the statement surgical goal but no guarantee affixed to the diagram or drawing and possibly initialed by the patient.

---

210 This relates to the mle that the statute of limitations does not begin to mn until the the time of the discovery ..

168

Claims of medical negligence have been dropped or dismissed because of the patient's failure to file the suit within the period of time defined by the statute of limitations. The documentation of date and time that the patient was advised of the circumstances of the injury have been crucial in preventing these claims from being pursued.

Managing a Claim

Notify Carrier

Dissatisfied patients, particularly those who have suggested, through action or attitude, that they are considering legal action, must be reported to the physician's medical-liability carrier. The carrier must also be immediately notified if the patient or an attorney requests a copy of medical records regarding the patient or if the patient and/or an attorney asks for a meeting to fully discuss the medical care rendered and the results obtained. A physician should never meet with an attorney regarding the care rendered to a patient in which there may be a potential negligence claim without notifying and receiving approval from the insured's carrier. The carrier must be notified if the physician receives a letter from an attorney that indicates a patient is considering filing a suit, or upon notification that a suit has been filed. If a physician considers that a significant potential for exposure to a medical negligence claim exists, the carrier should be advised.

A physician who assumes care as a treating physician for a patient who is filing suit against another physician may be contacted by a plaintiffs attorney who asks for an appointment to discuss the patient's condition. Even though the second physician may appear to have no claim exposure, his own liability carrier should be contacted and advised of the attorney's request for the following reasons:

Exposure could exist of which the second physician is unaware. A conference with a plaintiff's attorney may provide that attorney with information to that effect that might later prove detrimental to the second physician.

The second physician may be covered by the same liability carrier as the physician against whom the suit is being filed. In cases where one policy holder may provide information to a plaintiff's attorney that might prove detrimental to another policy holder, the carrier may wish to have a defense attorney present.

Secure and Organize All Records on the Patient

If a claim seems imminent, locate and organize all the patient's records. Immediately, copies should be made of all records, and the original placed in a secure location to prevent accidental loss or unintentional alteration. Do not make any changes in any records or charts. Do not dispose of any records, x-rays, photographs, or any other material that relate to the patient, whether it be medical or nonmedical.

In assisting the defense attorney, the defendant may create additional notes and narratives to make the written record more understandable. In no instance, should these notes or additions be brought to formal hearings such as depositions or the trial itself. Such notes and information are usually considered "privileged" (i.e., protected by the attorney/client privilege) and are not subject to discovery except when they are brought to formal hearings. Each page containing information pertaining to the claim, but which is not in the patient's records, should be headed by the written statement: "personal communication to my attorney" (insert the defense attorney's name if possible).

Review only materials approved) by the defense attorney, one's own records, and the hospital records, in order to avoid exposing oneself to new areas of inquiry.

Do Not Discuss the Case with Anyone

Do not discuss the case with anyone besides the carrier and defense attorney. Plaintiff's attorneys, through interrogatories and depositions, will ask the identity of any individual with whom the defendant physician has discussed the case. The plaintiff's attorney will then ask these individuals about the conversations, in hopes of finding some variation or inconsistency in the physician's sworn testimony as compared to the dialogue that may have occurred with others. Discussion about the case among codefendants can suggest the appearance of "collusion" and should be avoided unless expressly approved by the defense attorney.

Prepare to Invest Time

Medical liability claims frequently involve months of preparation and, if the claim progresses, the trial may not occur for several years after it has been filed. The defendant physician must be prepared to invest time in a review of the facts of the case and provide assistance to the defense attorney regarding details that might not be contained in the medical records. Interrogatories must be answered and depositions scheduled that will require significant preparation on the part of the defendant physician. In addition, the defendant physician may be asked to attend depositions taken from other parties involved in the suit, most notably those of the plaintiff and the plaintiff's expert. The plaintiff may choose experts from other cities or states. Attending such depositions may result in considerable inconvenience, expense, and time away from one's practice.

On the road to trial, pretrial conferences and reviews will occur that require additional tine. If the claim involves several defendants, additional conferences may be scheduled by the respective defense attorneys so as to better understand each defendant's exposure. If the case proceeds to trial, the trial may last days to weeks. Each day of testimony may be followed by additional conferences to assess the testimony and its effect on the physician's defense.

"Maneuvering" is a way of life in the legal profession. Scheduled depositions that necessitate the cancellation of a day of practice can be canceled by the attorney with little or no notice. As the time investment in the legal process becomes greater and greater, and the time available to practice medicine becomes less and less, defendant physicians become increasingly more willing to settle claims, even those that seem to have little or no merit. Initially, the physician may feel that the medical-liability claim is an assault on the physician's competence, professional skill, and integrity. As the suit drags on, the physician may come to the realization that the greatest threat in a medical-liability claim is in terms of lost time - precious time spent away from patients.

Assist the Defense Attorney

The defense attorney handling the defendant physician's case will, most often, be an expert in the management of medical negligence claims. The attorney may not be familiar with procedures, surgical indications, and other details associated with the medical treatment provided in the defendant's case. It is the obligation of the defendant physician to provide the necessary background material and understanding of medical treatment so that the defense attorney is enabled to develop an effective defense.

The defendant physician must be prepared to dedicate whatever time is required to do this effectively and completely.

It will be the plaintiff's contention that the defendant physician failed to act in accordance with the prevailing standard of care. The attorney will argue that the defendant failed to utilize the degree of knowledge, care, and skill which would have been exercised by another similarly qualified physician under the same or similar circumstances. The defense attorney must be provided with the necessary medical information to determine if, in fact, there exists a deviation from the standard of care. The defendant physician knows much of this information. It is the defendant's responsibility to convey this information to the defense attorney. Honesty and candor are absolutely essential, and failure to convey all pertinent medical facts and information (even though they may appear unfavorable) will significantly diminish the attorney's ability to understand the case and develop an effective defense. The defendant physician will be asked to provide the names of "experts" who are familiar with the medical discipline in question and who would be willing to review the case. The experts must provide an opinion as to the applicable standard of care and an opinion as to whether a deviation from that standard caused the plaintiffs injury.

The defense of medical-liability claims is a specialty within the practice of law, very much as plastic surgery is a specialty within the practice of medicine. The proper management of a medical-liability claim requires a specialized attorney. The defendant must rely upon the expertise of the attorney if any success is to be expected in the defense. Peculiarities of defending medical negligence claims may only be known to attorneys specializing in this area and may not be easily understood by the defendant physician. It is important that the defendant rely upon the attorney's advice in matters relating to legal theory and the defense strategies most appropriate for the circumstances.

With the increase in the numbers of medical negligence claims, defense attorneys are frequently involved in the defense of more than one case. The attorney's enthusiasm for each case may be significantly tempered by the defendant physician's enthusiasm, cooperation, and willingness to assist. Defendant physicians who demonstrate an indifference, lack of concern, and an unwillingness to invest the necessary time and effort for the development of an appropriate defense may be in danger of generating similar attitudes in the defense attorney.

Interrogatories

Depositions

A deposition, or examination before trial (EBT), is part of the legal process called *discovery*. The defendant physician is examined in order to establish the defendant's position with regards to the treatment rendered, as well as to allow the plaintiff to learn new factual avenues to investigate.[211] Depositions are usually restricted to obtaining testimony from the named parties and from the experts who will testify at trial.

Physicians may consider the trial the focal point of any medical negligence action. Attorneys, rather, consider the depositions to be of greater importance. To a plaintiff's attorney, the single most important deposition is that of the defendant physician. Many medical negligence claims are significantly influenced by the defendant physician's deposition and therefore physicians must not underestimate the importance of the testimony to be given at this examination. Deposition preparation is very much like board preparation. The defendant physician must be informed, knowledgeable, and familiar with the treatment rendered as well as with all pertinent medical records, x-rays, test results, the medical literature, and any additional data that has been gleaned through discovery and investigation during the claim's course.

The answers provided during the deposition will, in essence, freeze such testimony and "etch it in stone". Every question asked has a purpose that relates to the matter at hand. Answers must be precise, audible, accurate, appropriately qualified, and clearly understandable, so there can be no misinterpretation of the question or the answer later at trial. Simple gestures without audible responses are unacceptable. The testimony, once established, is used as the basis for both plaintiff and defense attorneys for trial preparation.

---

211 Alton WG Jr. *Malpractice: a trial lawyer's advice for physicians.* Boston: Little, Brown, 1977; 14.8.

Deposition testimony may hold more weight than trial testimony, because depositions are usually taken well in advance of trial and therefore are closer in time to the events in question. Corrections or changes in testimony at the time of trial, when compared to deposition testimony, will be characterized by the attorney as a reflection of the fact that the defendant was coached or is changing the answers to avoid liability.

Depositions are conducted under oath, outside the courtroom, usually in one of the attorney's offices. The defendant physician must remember that testimony is being provided for informational purposes and not for the justification of treatment. No judge or jury is present to decide whether the defendant is guilty of medical negligence.

The purpose of the defendant physician's deposition, from the plaintiff's point of view, is to:

Obtain information.

Test the defendant as a witness and determine the positive or negative qualities the physician may possess that would make either a favorable or unfavorable jury impression.

Develop inconsistencies and illicit damaging statements from the defendant under oath that might later be used to discredit him or her.

Deposition testimony differs from trial testimony. The purpose of the deposition is discovery. While answers should be as complete as necessary to prevent misinterpretation, they should also be concise and confined as closely as possible to the scope of the question. *Information must not be volunteered when it is not essential to answering the question.* To do so may provide information that was new ground," which will not only lengthen the deposition but also may provide information that may be detrimental.

Do not guess! If the precise details or information cannot be recalled, the defendant physician (deponent) should answer "I do not remember." If, during the course of events the answer to the question is remembered or if information is later obtained to provide that answer, it may later be possible to explain at trial that the deponent's memory was refreshed and accurate testimony can then be provided. However, if the deponent has already taken a position on the basis of a guess at deposition, the testimony cannot be changed at trial without the risk of being discredited.

In answering questions, the deponent must consider every factor relevant to the answer and then reach a positive and unequivocal response. Physicians possess scientific minds, and in the desire for absolute truth many physicians tend to equivocate when answering. In the jurors' minds, equivocation conjures negative implications and resultant disbelief.

The attorney must not be permitted to summarize the defendant's testimony in the attorney's own words and then ask for confirmation. The defendant should always answer in his own words so as to avoid contradiction with previous testimony. If a question is asked about documented evidence, the document must be reviewed completely before answering. Deponents must watch for leading questions from attorneys that provide a set of facts that are only partly true, which then place the witness in conflict with previous testimony. If a legitimate mistake is made during deposition, it can be corrected before trial.

The defense attorney may play a very passive role during the deposition that is conducted by the plaintiff's attorney. The defense attorney is present to protect the defendant but doesn't wish to disclose facts or opinions of which the plaintiffs attorney is unaware or divulge information that may reveal the defense strategy.

Trial

Most medical negligence claims do not reach trial. As additional facts and data are obtained through discovery and investigation, the evidence will either influence the plaintiff to drop the suit or influence the defendant to settle. However, claims in which the plaintiff believes the evidence supports the contention that the defendant was negligent and when the offers of settlement (if any) by the defendant are not sufficient to compensate for the injury, the claim will go to trial. Conversely, if the defendant believes that there was no negligence and the plaintiff refuses to drop the suit, the claim will go to trial.

The actual trial may not occur for years after its filing, and a considerably longer time will have elapsed from the time that the alleged negligent act occurred. By the time of trial, the defendant physician will be well acquainted with the facts of the case and with the position of the other principals, including the defense attorney, plaintiff, plaintiff's attorney, and the defense and plaintiff experts. The defendant will have had the opportunity to study the deposition given by the various parties to the suit, including his or her own deposition. The defense attorney, in cooperation with the defendant, will have established the theory and defense plan.

For the well prepared defendant, the trial should be a relatively atraumatic experience, but most physician defendants indicate that trial experience is anything but benign. The courtroom is the legal profession's "operating room." This legal setting can generate the same anxieties for the physician defendant that a surgical suite generates for a patient. In addition to being prepared regarding the facts of the case, the defendant must also be prepared to be a courtroom "figure," whose manner and demeanor will be on display throughout trial and can influence the success or failure of the defense.

Attitudes that project indifference, arrogance, or condescension must be avoided. The defendant must appear concerned, sincere, knowledgeable, and sympathetic.

When testifying as a witness, answers should be provided in a straightforward manner. If the answer is yes or no, the defendant should respond accordingly and avoid trying to expand or evade. Such a self-serving stance will negatively impress the jury. At trial, unlike deposition, testimony must stand the test of a cross-examination in order to permit the jury to judge the witness' credibility. Leading, argumentative, and loaded questions are attempted in cross-examination, whereas such questions would not be broached during a deposition.

The defendant's attention must be directed to the proceedings at all times to reinforce and project the impression of the defendant's concern and interest, but also to enable the defendant physician to assist the defense attorney in matters of fact with regard to medical testimony as it is presented.

The defense attorney will manage events occurring during the trial and will guide the physician defendant accordingly. Much of the proceedings are beyond the control or influence of the defendant physician. This can be quite frustrating for a person who is used to "taking charge." The defendant must largely assume a passive role in the proceedings and rely upon the expertise and experience of the defense attorney.

Other Medical-Legal Encounters

TESTIMONY AS A TREATING PHYSICIAN NOT PARTY TO A SUIT

A physician may be asked to give a deposition regarding treatment of a patient in support of a patient's claim against another party (e.g., in an auto accident, regarding another physician defendant, regarding a manufacturer in a products liability case, or in actions to establish disability compensation). If the physician's testimony might raise a question of medical negligence as to his treatment of the patient, the physician's insurance company should be advised. The insurance company may wish to have an attorney present during the deposition to advise and protect the treating physician.

When testifying as a treating physician of a patient who is bringing suit against another doctor, the treating physician is required only to provide factual information pertaining to treatment. An opinion as to whether the previous physician deviated from the standard of care must be obtained from an "expert" (even though the treating physician may qualify as an expert). If asked to give an opinion as to whether the defendant physician deviated from the standard of care, the treating physician may properly respond "I have no opinion." If, however, the treating physician chooses to give an opinion, that opinion will almost certainly have to be repeated at trial.

EXPERTS

The essential question in medical negligence claims is whether the treatment deviated or departed from the accepted standard of practice. Such a determination will depend on what the expert witnesses testify is the accepted standard or practice under the circumstances. Usually, before a plaintiffs attorney accepts a case, the attorney will ask for a case review by an expert physician, often a physician whom the attorney has used in the past as a consultant. Defense attorneys use consultants in the same capacity. Upon review of the case, the consultant will provide an oral report to the attorney about whether evidence exists that the treating physician deviated from the standard of care. Consultants are not obligated to testify as experts unless they agree to do so. If the plaintiff's attorney accepts the case, expert testimony will have to be provided that supports the plaintiff's contention that the treatment rendered deviated from the accepted standards. Similarly, the defendant must also provide an expert to support the defendant's position that no deviation existed. If the consultants do not wish to serve as experts, the attorneys must obtain other experts who are willing to appear for deposition called by the opposing party and who are willing to be called as trial expert witnesses by the party paying for the experts' services.

Since jurors have no independent knowledge with which to judge the quality of care as compared to the accepted standards, the testimony of the experts is crucial in the decision of the case. The weight that jurors assign to expert testimony will depend on such factors as (a) the witness' demeanor, background, and qualifications, as well as general persuasiveness; (b) the ability of the witness to hold up under cross-examination; (c) the credibility of the opposing expert testimony; (d) the demeanor of the opposing expert; and (e) such intrinsic evidence as the medical records, x-rays, and laboratory tests, not to mention (f) the testimony of the parties and other witnesses.

Because of the pivotal importance of expert testimony in a medical negligence case, expert witnesses are usually subjected to strenuous cross-examination. The expert's qualifications in terms of training, teaching positions, hospital affiliations, contributions to the literature, and the like, add weight to the expert's opinion. Equally or even more important is the manner in which the expert states the opinion. The opinions expressed must be unequivocal and definitive. If an expert opinion is too speculative and the expert appears unsure, the testimony will usually carry no weight with the jurors.

Defendants, as well as expert witnesses, have to deal with expert questions posed in various forms.[212] One of the most dramatic is the long hypothetical question in which the interrogator asks the witness to "assume" certain facts to be true. If the witness disagrees with the truth of the assumptions contained in the hypothetical question, the witness may respond that the question cannot be answered because some of the assumptions stated in the question are not true. If the interrogating attorney insists that the witness assume their truth, the witness should respond: "If everything you asked me to assume were true, which I disagree with and find unlikely, my opinion would be ... "

212 Alton WG Jr. *Malpractice: a trial lawyer's advice for physicians.* Boston: Little, Brown, 1977; 203.

When providing an expert opinion, the witness should also note all the relevant reasoning and data that led to the opinion. Doing so not only demonstrates the expert's knowledge of the medicine involved and of the case but also lends credence to the expert's opinion in the eyes of the jury.

Opposing attorneys will often attempt to impeach the opinions of an expert witness on cross-examination by introducing the contrary opinion of a published authority. This tactic requires the use of medical literature. To do so, the witness must recognize the publication as authoritative, or its author as an authority in the field. If the work or the author is not recognized by the witness as authoritative, the cross-examining attorney is not permitted to use the contrary opinion to impeach the expert witness' opinion. An expert is not compelled to recognize any publication or author, no matter how widely used or famous.[213] If the witness feels that a certain text must be acknowledged as authoritative, the answer may still be qualified by a statement to the effect that the witness still does not agree with all the opinions expressed in the text. If, in an attempt to embarrass an expert who refuses to accept any text as authoritative, the cross-examining attorney introduces a large number of texts in an effort to make the witness appear unfamiliar with the literature, the witness should indicate awareness of the existence of the work but not accept it as being authoritative and give reasons.

DEFENSIBLE MEDICAL RECORDS

"If it wasn't charted, it wasn't done."

Every medical professional has heard that phrase so often it's become axiomatic. Is it true? Of course not. Physicians make mistakes in the chart; they get very busy and may forget to document certain information; and they may sometimes deliberately omit certain information.

---

213 Ibid.,

The axiom would seem to have a corollary: if it was charted it was done. Is this true? No more than the original saying. Most physicians can remember reading medical records and seeing entries that are questionable or don't make sense. On occasion these entries have been made in error (i.e., the event or treatment occurred but was documented in the wrong patient's chart); sometimes they have even been made in a deliberate attempt to falsify the record.

What role does the medical record serve?[214]

Although not primarily a legal document, if admitted in court it serves as a legal document to represent the quality of care, or to prove the extent of a patient's injuries.

It serves as a communication channel among members of the health care team.

It provides evidence for evaluating the quality of care.

It provides evidence for determining eligibility for third party payments.

It's a source of information about communicable diseases.

In the event of a malpractice suit, it serves as the record of what actually happened during the course of a patient's treatment.

It documents the actual quality of care rendered, which m turn contributes or detracts from quality in perception.

In a malpractice case, the medical record will be the first point of offense for the plaintiff and the first point of defense for the defendant, as noted in the next section on "Handling Malpractice Litigation." Therefore, it may be useful to start with the characteristics of a defensible chart and examine how the medical record is used by both defense and plaintiffs' attorneys.

Characteristics of the Defensible Medical Record

It is useful to consolidate the characteristics of the defensible medical record into a mnemonic device: LAWSUIT. Each letter stands for one or more characteristics which contribute to your defense.[215]

---

214 Tomes JP. *Compliance guide to electronic health records: a practical guide to legislation, codes, regulations and industry standards.* Faulker&Gray, 1994.
215 Tuthill E.I., *Medical staff documentation.* Tampa, FL, 1994.

Legible. As noted above, the medical record is a means of communication. If it can't be read, it can't "communicate." It's axiomatic that doctors have notoriously poor handwriting. Not only is it important that the record be legible in case it is admitted into evidence, it's also important that consultants be able to read your writing if they evaluate or treat your patient. If you choose transcription, make sure you read the transcribed record. Failure to read it may be considered negligence, since it may contain errors that only you could catch.

Since the record serves as a means of communication among members of the health care team, it must be in a form that makes communication easy. If your writing is poor, dictate your entries and have them transcribed. If you don't read it, and someone else - a nurse, another physician - relies on erroneous information, you could be liable.

Accurate. Be specific in what you write. Vague terms like "excessive", "severe" or "somewhat" present problems, not only for a legal team but also for the medical team. Terms such as those mean different things to different people. Indeed, even though you know today what you mean by writing "Severe bleeding noted", your sense of the term may have changed in five or six years when you are on the witness stand explaining your notes to a jury. Further, if a hostile expert gives his interpretation of what your terms mean, you can be sure that his or her testimony will put you in a bad light.

Also under the "accurate" heading comes the characteristic of objectivity. The record should contain only your objective professional impressions: what you see, hear, feel, and smell. Your personal impressions are also permitted unless they are peripheral to clinical issues or the quality of care. For example, if two physicians differ on their opinions regarding treatment for the same patient, they should document their opinion and not make "sidebar" comments about the other. The same is true of your personal opinions about the patient, the patient's family, and other members of the health care team. In short, if the comment, observation, or entry you wish to make has to do with clinical issues and direct care of the patient, go ahead and make the entry in objective terms. If the comment or observation is peripheral to the patient's care, don't put it in the medical record.

In addition to precision and objectivity, the "accurate" caveat extends to the need to avoid self-serving statements. Tuthill[216] tells of a record which stressed that a delivery was done "very carefully", with a breech extraction being performed "gently and very carefully". The infant whose delivery was described was found to be suffering from a fracture of the right forearm, which likely was sustained during birth. The self-serving verbiage was a red flag to the claims examiner, who was familiar with the physician's usual style and found the wording suspicious.

Whole. The record should be complete. Of course, missing pages or documents create "red flags" for attorneys. Beyond that, the record should tell a story, starting with the disposition. In between there should appear a logical series of events that account for everything that happened to the patient.

Therefore, the record should include:

Complete history and all physicals.

The patient's reason for seeking treatment.

Present clinical status of symptoms, organs and extremities.

Past history of relevant medical happenings.

Working diagnosis or differential diagnosis.

Admission notes.

Discharge summary.

Complete medication chart.

Physician progress notes.

Nursing notes.

Record of lab and radiology test ordered.

Lab and radiology reports and results.

IV flow sheets, respiratory and physical therapy notes.

Operative reports.

Informed consent.

---

216 Ibid.

Not all of these records are under the direct control of the individual physician. However, the medical staff, through its committee structure (i.e., executive committee, quality review committee, etc.), can periodically assess the completeness of charts and recommend changes, if any are needed.

In your office records, the same principles apply. Be especially careful to include documentation of phone conversations with or about patients. Although doctors (and their staffs) frequently talk with patients or family members on the phone, it's too seldom that those calls are documented in the medical record.

There are various formats for medical records, including:

The source-oriented record, in which physician notes, nurses' notes, lab reports, etc. are filed in separate sections.

The problem-oriented medical record, which includes minimum data on each patient, a problem list, initial plans and progress notes.

The integrated plan, which simply arranges records in a chronological order.

One final note about the "whole" aspect of medical record keeping: sign all your entries! This goes for office charts as well as hospital charts and holds true for your assistants who make entries. It's not uncommon to see unsigned entries made by staff members who haven't worked for the doctor for months or years; and there's no way to tell who is responsible for making the entry.

Substantiated. As indicated above, the medical record should tell a story. Further, your thought processes should substantiate what you do with the patient. For example, if a patient presents to her family physician with symptoms of fatigue, nausea, tenderness in the abdomen and aching joints, the physician may consider a number of diseases and test for any or all of them. However, if the doctor considered hepatitis B, but did not test for it, he should be prepared to substantiate his or her reasoning.

One medical-legal expert notes that it's very easy to tell when a physician thinks he or she has a problem with the management of a specific patient. "Two weeks of one-line progress notes become full paragraphs, with extensive explanations for what's being done and what isn't being done. It's obvious that something has happened.

It will also be obvious to a plaintiffs attorney and certainly to a medical expert. The solution? Substantiate before you get into trouble."[217]

Substantiation is useful for staying out of court, but it's also useful in the courtroom. A jury will look to your chart for evidence that supports what you are saying. If the evidence isn't there, you may well be in trouble. The plaintiff's medical expert will likely presume you didn't know what you were doing, or will presume you were wrong.

Remember, when you substantiate your reasoning you're doing "defensive documentation". On the other hand, selecting a course of treatment which excludes others is dangerous if you don't write down why you're doing what you're doing. Keep in mind this step is not only for you today; it's for you years in the future if you are pressed to explain why you did or didn't take a particular course of action.

The SOAP format is a good means of substantiating what you do. By documenting the subjective (what the patient says/ chief complaint), objective (what the physician sees, hears, and measures), assessment (what the physician thinks is going on with the patient) and plan (what he or she intends to do about it), the physician is creating a logical thought process that stands up well in court.

Unaltered. An improper alteration can eliminate the medical record from evidence. That's not to the physician's benefit: the record is the best evidence, and often the only evidence. To lose it because of an improper alteration is unfortunate.

Illegal alterations cause problems not only for your case in a lawsuit, but also for your career and pocketbook. Illegal alterations frequently result in punitive damages. An Illinois pediatrician paid $5.000,000 in punitive damages because he altered a record; a Kansas OB paid $1.9 million for altering fetal monitoring strips. Who paid? The physicians - punitive damages, by law, are not covered by insurance.

---

217 Ibid.

184

Alterations also may result in charge of fraud being brought against the offending physician. This is a serious charge which may cause a physician to lose his or her license, as well as invalidate the physician's professional liability insurance.

If you do make an error, it's all right to change an entry, as long as it's done in an acceptable manner. What's acceptable? The recommended manner is to draw a single line through the part to be corrected; write the word "error" above the line, with your initials and the date of the change; and below the error make the corrected entry. Variations of this technique are acceptable, within reason. Some hospitals have their own procedures for correcting medical records. The key is to make the change in such manner that the original entry is still legible, thereby showing that you are not trying to cover up or hide what was originally there. The issue at trial will be to distinguish between a legitimate error or an intentional cover-up. Be sure your corrections show that you didn't mean to mislead the reader.

What if you notice an error in someone else's entry? Don't correct it yourself. Go ahead and make your entry as you normally would, then discuss the incorrect entry with the person who made it. If the entry is not an error, but simply a difference of opinion, it can be noted as such objectively without pointing fingers at the other party. For example: "Nurse's note of 3:00 p.m. read. My findings are as follows: ... ". That way, you let it be known that you read the other entry and have acted appropriately.

Late entries are acceptable, too, within reason, as long as they are dated on the date the entry is actually made. Never date a late entry as though it were being made when it should have been made originally. Doing so is a conscious attempt to falsify the record, and will render it indefensible if caught.

How late is too late to make a late entry? Most hospitals have policies that specify time frames for making late entries and completing charts. In general, if the patient is still in the hospital, it's permissible. Consider, however, the effect of a late entry on a jury. For example, if you warn a patient about possible side effects of medication but don't write that in your progress notes, and the patient suffers the side effects and is injured, resist the temptation to go back and make a late entry noting your original warning. Doing so after the patient has already been injured will look defensive and put you in a bad light for a jury. You would be better off testifying that you did, in fact, give the warning and didn't write it down. If you can do so persuasively and come across as a sympathetic, caring doctor who was doing the right thing, you'll be much better off than if you made the defensive late entry. It has been pointed out that there is a direct 1:1 correlation between altered records and successful plaintiffs.[218]

The danger of altering records is illustrated by a case involving a family physician. He treated a 12-year old boy for knee pain and referred the patient to an orthopedic surgeon for evaluation. The orthopedist told the patient's parents that the problem should have been treated much earlier. Several months later, the family physician received official notice of intent to sue. He looked at the record and noted that he had not documented the referral to the orthopedist and made a late entry in a manner designed to make it look like the referral had been charted at the time of the patient's last visit. Unfortunately for the doctor, his staff had already given the patient's parents a copy of the original unaltered record. When the plaintiffs attorney reviewed the two versions it was apparent that there was an attempt to deceive. The case was indefensible and settled out of court.

Intelligible. As previously noted, other members of the health care team rely on the record to make decisions about the patient's care. They must be able to carry out your orders and provide good care, based on what you have documented.

Use only approved abbreviations, keeping in mind that some abbreviations carry dual meanings even within the same facility. For example, "LOC" may be interpreted either as "level/loss of consciousness" or as "laxative of choice." You may have developed your own shorthand over the years, but should resist the temptation to use it in the record. It may make perfect sense to you, but baffle others who need to understand what you've written.

Timely. Most physicians are prompt with their office notes, but may lag in their hospital charts. Remember, the longer you wait the more you forget. Your perception changes as well, and you may be inclined to omit key information that should be included.

---

218 Ibid.

Tuthill tells of a plaintiffs attorney who requested a copy of the hospital record months after the patient had been discharged. The medical record department noticed that the chart was incomplete, and notified the physician to complete the chart as soon as possible. The doctor, fearing a lawsuit, dictated a lengthy discharge summary which put himself in the best possible light. On reviewing the chart the plaintiff's attorney read the self-serving remarks, and noted that the discharge summary had been dictated months after discharge - indeed, after the attorney had requested the records. If the attorney can convince the court that the discharge note was made after an umeasonably long delay, the court may be willing to exclude the note from evidence, thus eliminating the evidence that clearly established the patient's condition on discharge.[219]

Be sure to note the time you make each entry. This is true for both office and hospital charts. It's advisable to use a single clock as your guide - in the hospital, the clock on the wall in the ER or at the nurse's station; in your office, the clock on the wall in the exam room or at the reception desk. Why? It's common for timepieces to be at variance with each other. In the hospital, for example, if the triage nurse states that the physician was called at 11 :45 p.m., and the doctor writes that he first examined the patient at 12:02, there will be a question about those missing 17 minutes. In reality, the nurse may have called the doctor at 11:49, and he arrived to examine the patient at 11 :53, but because both used their wristwatches (which were off a few minutes) the variance seemed much more significant.

Protecting Patient Records

Some traditional concerns about medical record handling and security include:

-Releasing originals.

-Charging too much for copies.

-Denying a patient his records because of an outstanding bill.

-Confusing the records of patients with similar names.

-Keeping non-clinical documents (insurance correspondence, legal or malpractice related correspondence, etc.) together with clinical documents in the medical record.

---

219 Ibid.

-Destroying or discarding records when you believe they are no longer needed.

Management of Risk Factors

Always keep original medical records in your possession. The patient has a right to the information in the record, but the record itself is the physician's property.

If patient records are subpoenaed, the requesting attorney should obtain his client's written consent for release and give it to you. However, before you release the information, the patient or authorized representative is required to give the physician written authorization to disclose confidential information.[220] You have the right to insist on proof of this before providing the records.

If the patient requests a copy of his chart, a copy should be provided. You can charge a reasonable amount for the copies. What's reasonable? Also, do not deny a patient copies of his medical record because he has an outstanding bill. His right to the records supersedes his financial status with you.

Make sure records are all organized consistently. There are various filing systems which are appropriate; just don't mingle two or more.

Have an "alert" system to warn you of potential name similarities. One such system is to stamp in red ink "NAME ALERT" on the chart's cover and first page, then to cross-reference the patient by birth date, social security number, or other identifying key.

Non-clinical information such as billing records or documents necessary only for reimbursement or federal or state health programs should not be included in the patient record. Keep them separate, either in separate files or in a separate section apart from clinical information within the medical record file. In some states in the USA this is statutory.[221]

All malpractice-related correspondence or notations of conversations between physician, other health care provider, and malpractice carrier should be kept separate from either medical or financial records. Never make an entry in the medical record regarding conversations with attorneys about malpractice suits.

---

220 Ibid.
221 Tomes JP. *Compliance guide to electronic health records: a practical reference to legislation, codes, regulations and industry standards.* New York, Faulkner&Gray, 1994, p. 4.

Although some states have laws permitting destruction of medical records after a certain period of time, from a risk management standpoint you should keep the records forever. If that presents some physical or logistical problems, put them on microfilm or use a bonded off-site storage facility. You can't predict when you may need to refer back to a record of a patient you last treated twenty years ago. If that record is important, you need to be able to review it, to protect yourself and the patient.

Exercise: Finding the Risks

You are reviewing a patient's chart in the hospital and notice that a resident wrote an order for a medication to which your patient is allergic. The allergy is noted in the history, but apparently was overlooked. The incorrect medication should have been given an hour ago, but due to fluctuations in nursing staffing patterns it wasn't given.

How many risk management issues are present in this scenario? How would you handle them? See discussion on below.

Discussion: Finding the Risks

There are multiple risks in this hypothetical scenario. A few:

Why did the resident write an order without first checking the patient's allergies? If s/he did so after a cursory look at the medication sheet where no allergy was noted, the resident clearly breached his or her duty to the patient. It is the physician\s responsibility to make sure that medications are prescribed and appropriately administered. The fact that the allergy prominently flagged on the chart doesn't absolve the physician from responsibility.

Why was the allergy not noted more prominently? Most hospitals have a procedure for "flagging" allergies in red, or noting them prominently on the medication sheet, or on the front of the medical record. If this hospital had such a procedure and a glitch in the system caused the allergy to be omitted, the hospital has breached its duty. If it didn't have such a procedure, it still breached its duty, because the standard of care calls for such a procedure.

What should the physician do about the incorrect medication order? Is it proper for him to correct another physician's written order? Technically, the answer is "no" - he shouldn't correct another doctor's order. A preferable course of action would be for our physician to contact the physician who made the erroneous order and suggest that it be corrected immediately. In the meantime he or she could write a new order, with a note that the correction was made to accommodate the patient's allergy. The new order should be signed by the physician who writes it.

Also, the nurses and medical records staff need to know about the problem. This is best done through the quality assurance/quality improvement process.

8. HANDLING MALPRACTICE LITIGATION

If you are targeted in a malpractice lawsuit, don't panic. The course of a suit isn't pleasant, but knowing what to expect, what the plaintiffs' attorneys may be doing, and how to handle each step can make it easier.

After the Adverse Event

Before a suit is filed there must occur some type of medical misadventure that would prompt a patient to seek out the services of a plaintiff's attorney. Since these misadventures may be minor as well as major, whenever something happens that you don't expect, pay particular attention to patient/family relations and documentation. Make sure you document facts, observations, and differential diagnoses on a routine basis. This will be helpful in proving you carefully considered the case and your course of action. When you record a diagnosis, state in the record other possibilities that you considered but ruled out, as suggested in the previous section on medical record documentation. Do not attempt to alter a prior note after the adverse event. Doing so may eliminate any chance of a valid defense.

Tempted to write a personal note and keep it in your secret file at home? Remember: personal notes or narrative dictation for your personal records cannot be protected from discovery and therefore should not be made. If there is something important enough to record, it either belongs in the chart or in a confidential letter to an attorney that will not be discoverable. If a suit is filed, you will be asked for copies of every document you have that pertains to the patient, including medical records, billing records, and personal records. If you have made such personal notes and hold them back, you may be in contempt of court.

Keep communication lines open with patient and family. Tell them what happened, talking frankly in terms they can understand. Take the time to explain, and above all, don't avoid the family. Doing so may be interpreted as a sign of avoidance and guilt and will only add fuel to the fire.

How Plaintiffs' Attorneys Plan Their Strategy

Plaintiffs' attorneys have written extensively about planning medical malpractice cases. Here's an overview of how they work:

When a potential plaintiff first makes contact with the plaintiffs attorney, the contact (usually a phone call) is screened by a reviewer trained in medical malpractice law. This reviewer, who may or may not be a nurse, will ask targeted questions to determine the nature of the alleged fault, names of doctors and hospitals involved, and when the alleged fault happened. If the reviewer believes the case is worth pursuing further, the potential plaintiff is invited to come to the law office for an interview.[222] To that meeting the potential plaintiff is instructed to bring a chronology of the event, prior medical history of the patient involved, details regarding treatment and hospitalizations, billing records, and copies of any written materials that were received from the doctor or the hospital during the course of the event. The latter may be used to create a plaintiffs case for breach of contract, breach of warranty or deceptive trade practice. Some plaintiffs' attorneys also require that clients complete a comprehensive questionnaire, either before or at the initial meeting.[223] Finally, the potential client is asked to obtain a copy of the medical record (both hospital and office charts).

Contrary to what some physicians believe, plaintiffs' attorneys don't accept every case. They evaluate potential cases from a number of angles, considering questions such as:

Does the case have shock value? Some legal experts think that if the plaintiff's attorney isn't shocked by the case, then a jury won't be shocked either.[224] Examples of "shock value" cases include operating on the wrong body part, illegal alteration of records, members of the medical team lying to patients, etc. Fortunately, these types of events are relatively rare. Therefore, this isn't the sole criterion used in deciding whether to accept a case.

What kind of witness will the potential client make? If he or she (and family members) have poor memories, stammer, having difficult answering direct questions, the jury's impression will be less favorable. On the other hand, if the witnesses are sympathetic and would make a good impression, the plaintiff's attorney may be more willing to accept the case.

---

222 Turner JW. *Prosecuring a medical malpractice case.* Houston Law Review, Vol. 22:535, 1985.
223 Hamey OM, *supra*, p. 578.-587.
224 Ibid., p. 588

Potential damages. Plaintiffs' attorneys who specialize in medical malpractice expect to spend at least $5,000 out of pocket to develop a case, and advise that a case should be worth at least $100,000 in actual damages in order to take the case to trial.[225] Cases with less damages may still be accepted but likely will be presented for settlement, not trial.

What are the medical facts of the case? For this, the attorney will have the record reviewed by a medical consultant, usually a physician. The physician will offer an opinion about the case's worthiness. Plaintiffs' attorneys can access a wealth of literature on how to find medical experts. Further, they are coached in how to approach doctors to convince them to review cases and become expert witnesses.[226]

Some plaintiffs' attorneys advise against filing "iffy" cases. These cases, which have no more than a 50 percent chance of success, cost a lot to litigate and may well be lost at trial. These include cancer and cardiovascular cases, because the issue of causation is difficult for the plaintiff to prove; orthopedic cases based on trauma, because it is difficult to prove the physician, not the trauma, caused the problem; and postoperative infection cases, since it is difficult to prove what caused the infection.[227]

Once the case is accepted, the plaintiffs attorney will determine who to sue. There are usually multiple potential defendants, so factors like board certification, reputation, and malpractice insurance will play roles. Next, the attorney will file suit or send notice of intent to sue (see following section). With this notice will come a request for medical records. Records obtained from this request will be carefully compared with the records previously obtained by the client. Occasionally, there are discrepancies, which will probably be used against the defendant by the plaintiffs attorney.

The plaintiff's attorney has specific goals for deposition. Like the defense attorney, he wants to prepare for trial and reduce the risk of unpleasant surprises. He also wants to make the defense familiar with the facts of the case, which may induce the defense to settle.[228]

---

225 Shrager DS. *Screening and Preparing the Medical Negligence Case.* Trial, August, 1988, p. 16-20.
226 Laska L. *Malpractice experts:finding and using the best!* M.Lee Smith Publishers, Nashville, 1993.
227 trodel RC. *Securing and using medical evidence in personal injury and health-care cases.* Prentice-Hall, 1988, p.201-202
228 Harney, *supra*, p. 615

At deposition, the plaintiffs attorney will probably ask the defendant doctor to identify all persons involved in the case. This will help the plaintiffs target individuals they may have overlooked. The attorney may also ask the defendant physician to read his or her notes into the record. This will facilitate deciphering illegible notes and facilitate review by the plaintiff's expert.

Plaintiffs' attorneys like to videotape depositions when possible. Videotape shows when the defendant hesitates too long in answering, and also can show other signs of nervousness which may sway a jury.

After the deposition, the plaintiff's attorney will have the deposition reviewed by a medical expert. Sometimes they will find discrepancies that will benefit them at trial.

After discovery, both sides will take a good look at the possibility of settlement. Most plaintiffs prefer settlement, since trials are expensive, time-consuming, and usually won by the defendant physician.[229]

Notice of Pending Lawsuit

Some states require that a physician be given formal notice of pending suit before the actual suit is filed. If you receive a notice letter, do not respond with a substantive reply. Notify your insurer promptly. Don't prepare an unsolicited narrative or statement about the patient or the incident. Instead, wait for the insurer or your attorney to ask for that information. They know how to obtain information from you in a fashion that will be privileged. Also, don't add to, alter, or complete any incomplete portion of the chart after you've received a notice letter. By that time, chances are good that the original records are already in the hands of an attorney, and your modifications would be recognized immediately.

Never discuss any aspect of the case with anyone other than your insurer or your attorney. Such conversations are discoverable and very risky.

---

229 GAO, *Practitioner data bank: information on small medical malpractice payments.* July, 1992.

Regarding medical records, you will be required to provide complete and unaltered copies of the claimant's medical records to any requesting person who is party to the suit within provisions of your state laws as long as the request is accompanied by proper written authorization from the patient or his legal representative.

Do not release the original record. Release copies only. If the records are mailed, use certified mail with return receipt requested, so there is a record of the person receiving the records.

In some states, there is a waiting period to promote settlement of valid claims. Therefore, after you receive the notice letter, it is possible that no suit may be filed for a stated period. If the plaintiff does not abide by this rule, his suit is subject to abatement, not dismissal.

Per the conditions of your malpractice coverage, you must notify your insurer of your notice letter and possible suit. In addition, some policies require that you notify the insurer after an adverse event. Check under the "duties of insured" section of your policy to see if this applies to you.

All policies require that you cooperate in the defense of your claim. That means you must assist your attorney as required, attend depositions and trial, etc.

If you have excess coverage, don't rely on your primary carrier to notify the excess carrier. Do it yourself and obtain written acknowledgment from the carrier that it received your notice. Otherwise you may not be covered by the excess insurance.

Receipt of Suit Papers

You (or your attorney on your behalf) must respond to a suit m a timely manner as prescribed by law. Make a note of the answer date on your calendar immediately upon being served with suit papers, so you don't forget to respond. With your insurance company, confirm that an attorney has been hired and that an answer to your suit was filed in a timely manner.

Should you have a personal attorney? Although the insurance company will provide you with an attorney, you may want to retain a personal attorney. This is especially true if the suit involves potentially large liability. Your personal attorney will advise you and give you feedback on the performance of your insurer's counsel. The cost is usually modest in comparison with potential losses.

Discovery

Discovery is the pre-trial process by which each party obtains information about the case from the other party in order to prepare for trial.

As already mentioned, medical records are "discoverable", meaning they must be shared with the plaintiff. Most communication between you and your attorney is not discoverable, since it is considered privileged.

You will be subpoenaed for deposition, meaning your attorney will receive a legal document ordering you to appear at a certain time and place to give testimony. Subpoenas may also be used to compel your attendance at a trial or other pretrial proceeding.

Depositions are pre-trial proceedings at which witnesses are placed under oath to answer questions that are put to them by the attorneys in the case. Depositions are usually verbal, and recorded by a court reporter. Videotaped depositions are also becoming more common. When the plaintiff is being deposed, you should attend the deposition.

Here are some deposition tips from defense attorneys:

Don't guess or speculate.

Don't agree to generalities that really depend on the clinical picture.

Do take time to think before answering each question.

Don't answer just because you want to appear knowledgeable.

Don't volunteer on the basis of your assumption that you can convince the plaintiff's attorney that he made a mistake in suing you.

Do answer firmly and positively with respect to direct questions about the incident.

Avoid falling into the "if it wasn't charted, it wasn't done" trap. Plaintiffs' attorneys will most likely state or insinuate that your care was inadequate unless you state to the contrary in the chart. You can fight such insinuations but do so at the risk of becoming involved in a heated war of credibility, since there is no documentation to support what you assert.

Insist that your attorney prepare you adequately for deposition. Depending on your comfort level with the process, it could take a few hours to prepare, or it could take much longer. In any case, don't allow yourself to be talked into meeting with the attorney for only an hour or so pre-deposition to prepare. You deserve much better.

Interrogatories are written question-and-answer sessions, directed to other parties (not witnesses) in the suit. They are also answered under oath, and the answers may be used at trial. One party may serve a certain number of written questions to the other to be answered under oath. At trial, your answers may be read to the jury by the opposing party; therefore, your accurate and carefully-worded responses are critical. Don't let your attorney respond to interrogatories on your behalf. You should be closely involved.

Your involvement during discovery will probably be limited to answering written interrogatories from the plaintiffs attorney, producing medical records as directed, and having your deposition taken. If you are named in the suit, you're entitled to attend any proceedings you want, but be sure to work with your attorney and insurance carrier to do so.

Expert Testimony

Expert testimony is the means by which the "'standard of care" is established. The states regulate who may testify as an expert. In some states, for example, an expert witness must be practicing at the time he or she gives testimony, or at the time the claim arose; and must have knowledge of the accepted standards of medical care for the diagnosis, care, or treatment of the illness, injury or condition involved in the claim. However, the expert witness may not need to be from that state, or practice in a setting similar to that of the defendant. Alternatively, a person may qualify as an expert witness if the court so decides after a hearing conducted outside the presence of the jury.

Protecting Information From Discovery

As noted above, discovery is the process of finding out everything possible about a case. Some information is barred from discovery, meaning it's protected by law and must be kept confidential. Other types of information are discoverable, meaning it may be subpoenaed or otherwise introduced as evidence.

Therefore, it's important you understand the ramifications if you talk about the case with *anyone*.

You're usually safe from discovery when communicating with your attorney. Documents produced by your attorney as he or she works on your case are also protected from discovery. However, if someone else (not your attorney) works on the case (for example, your insurance claims department working independently from your attorney, or an investigator) those work products or communications may not be protected.

For specific recommendations about protecting your communication and activities from discovery, consult an attorney.

The Course of Litigation

Most malpractice cases are filed in state court in a district or trial court, with one judge presiding. At this level the defendant has the option of a jury trial. When the jury's verdict is rendered, the verdict may be accepted by both parties. Often the verdict is appealed to the next level, usually an intermediate level of court known as appeals courts or appellate courts, made of three or more judges. At this level, attorneys prepare briefs on the case and present them to the court. The judges review the briefs and may hear arguments, but there is no jury trial. The appeals court may affirm the trial court's jury verdict (say it stands as is); may reverse it (say it was wrong), and/or may remand it (send it back for a new jury trial). The action of the court will depend to a very great degree on technical points (for example, whether the original jury was allowed to consider certain evidence or whether the charge to the jury was phrased appropriately). The court will also rely heavily on precedent (decisions reached in similar cases by the same court or higher courts).

The holding of the appeals court may be appealed to the court of last resort, usually the state supreme court. The procedures are similar (briefs, arguments, no jury trial); but the decision is final.

Disposition of the Case

How long does it take for the case to reach disposition? Times vary but generally range from two to five years.[230] As you would expect, there are more open claims (claims that still haven't been resolved) in more recent years. The more complex the case, the longer it takes to settle or go to trial.

As the suit and discovery progresses, your attorney may attempt to have the suit dismissed by moving for summary judgment. This motion may be granted if the plaintiff doesn't have an expert witness willing to testify that your treatment was below the "standard of care".

Another alternative is to settle the case or have the case dismissed. The court can dismiss the case for want of prosecution or as a sanction for failure of the plaintiff to provide discovery. The plaintiff can also dismiss his own action, but will be limited in his options for refiling unless the case involves a minor.

Most cases that go to trial are tried by a twelve-person jury. In these cases, the jury determines both the question of liability and damages. These cases usually last from one to three weeks; and, except for emergencies, you should try to be present for the entire trial if you are named in the suit.

The case is assigned to a particular judge and courtroom. After the judge has familiarized himself with the facts of the case, the jury is selected from a panel of prospective jurors who have been called to jury duty.

Once the jury is selected, the plaintiffs attorney makes an opening statement about the case from his perspective. Your attorney then makes an opening statement from your viewpoint. Then, the presentation of oral testimony and documentary evidence is made. The plaintiff presents his evidence first, then rests. Next, your defense presents its case. The plaintiff has a chance to rebut your evidence. The plaintiff always has the first and last word, since he has the burden of proof.

---

230 *Professionol liability statistics for physicians practicing in Texas.* Texas State Board of Medical Examiners, 1999.

Remember, the plaintiff must prove the four elements of malpractice. In most cases he must bring expert testimony about the standard of care for physicians in the same or similar circumstances, must show that you failed to meet that standard, and that your failure to meet that standard was the cause of the plaintiff's injury and damages.

Mediation

Mediation is growing in popularity as a cost- and time-effective means of resolving medical malpractice disputes. Mediation is an informal, private method in which a neutral person, the mediator, aids the disagreeing parties in reaching a mutual agreement or resolution. There is no formal presentation of witnesses or evidence, as in a trial. The mediation session is usually attended by the parties, their attorneys, and the mediator.

Most mediators are trained in conflict resolution, but unlike a judge in a civil matter, do not take sides or make decisions. The mediator's goal is to assist all parties in solving their problem through negotiation. Therefore, the key to a successful mediation is the willingness of both parties to reach agreement, therefore avoiding a formal suit. Since the process is informal, a mediation can usually be completed in a day or less, depending upon the skill of the mediator and the willingness of the involved parties to compromise. A mediation session is private and confidential. The process is voluntary and non-binding.

The mediation process usually involves six distinct stages m a carefully designed process:[231]

Mediator's opening statement. The disputing parties are introduced, and the mediator explains the goals and rules of the mediation. Each side is encouraged to work cooperatively toward settlement.

Disputants' opening statements (sometimes called a general caucus). Each party presents, in synopsis, what the dispute is about, how it has affected them, and offer some general ideas for resolution. Interruptions are not allowed. One of the main points of a general caucus is to set up the means for communication. Both parties must think about what has been said, not just what they want to say. It's important to trust your attorney.

---

231 Lovenheim, Peter. *How Mediation Really Works.* Nolo Press, 1996.

200

Joint discussion. The mediator tries to get each party to discuss the issues presented in the opening statements.

Private caucuses. This is where the majority of discussions take place. Each party meets privately with the mediator, discussing the strengths and weaknesses of their position, and propose new options for settlement. The mediator will caucus with each side as many times as needed, or until it becomes apparent that a resolution cannot be achieved. The mediator is the communication filter.

Joint negotiation. The parties are brought together for direct negotiations. Both parties must weigh the risks to facilitate settlement and be willing to talk about the case with the mediator.

Closure. The final state of the process, during which the parties will put the provisions in writing, if they have reached agreement. If no agreement has been reached, the mediator will summarize the progress of the discussions.

Mediations are usually successful for a number of reasons:

The mediation environment is "safe". The mediator can control and direct dialogue, avoiding unproductive discussions. Concessions or proposals are shared only if they are likely to lead to settlement.

The mediator keeps both parties focused and productive.

Each party has the opportunity to educate the other.

All involved decision-makers are usually present.

Each side can offer proposals for settlement without appearing to give in. More options for settlement may be explored.

And, each party has the chance to look closely at their case and the results they could expect in court.

Disadvantages:

Mediation may not resolve the dispute.

One party may not be happy with the solution or outcome.

The parties may have to go to court anyway. Points to remember:

The mediation process is about real people with real problems, concerns. hurts, grief, and anger.

Try to decide what your objectives are. What do you want to accomplish?

An absence of communication between patient and physician can cause hard feelings which impede settlement. Take time to talk to your patient.

Solutions come from many perspectives and parties differ about expectations and outcomes.

Communication must be constructive. You are trying to enable communication and make it work. Don't attack the other side.

The way something is said, rather than what is said, will make a great deal of difference.

Don't bring up extraneous issues. Focus on the matter at hand. Be prepared for the mediation session:

Communicate clearly.

Obtain necessary information and share it with your attorney.

Provide the mediator with the information s/lie needs regarding the case. Include strengths and weaknesses, history, and any special considerations.

Plan. Think about what you will say, and who you will bring to the mediation with you.

Case study

The plaintiff was a 52-year-old man who presented to his local physician complaining of nausea, vomiting, and lower quadrant pain. The physician suspected appendicitis and referred the patient to a surgeon, who diagnosed gallbladder disease and removed the gallbladder. The patient was then referred to another surgeon. Neither surgeon considered appendicitis in the differential diagnosis, even though the pathology report was negative with regard to the removed gallbladder. The plaintiff's pain continued, his white cell count increased, and his abdomen became distended. Nevertheless, the defendant surgeons did not consider an exploratory laparotomy for one week. When the exploratory laparotomy was performed the surgeons noted the remains of the ruptured appendix and considerable necrotic tissue. The patient required three further debridement procedures and remained hospitalized for 41 days. He has since been hospitalized for related conditions three times. The plaintiff sued, alleging negligence in failing to diagnose appendicitis and in failing to recognize the ruptured appendix. During the course of discovery, the plaintiff requested documents including reports prepared by quality assessment nurses, infection control reports, and transmittals between departments. The hospital objected on the grounds that these documents were protected by peer review statute.[232]

Since peer review documents are generally privileged, do you think the court would grant the plaintiffs request? See below for discussion.

Discussion

The court ruled that the documents requested were prepared independently of the peer review process and therefore were not privileged. The only way they could be privileged is if they had been prepared exclusively for the peer review committee and never left the confines of the committee records. Since these reports were transmitted from department to department, via interoffice mail or by hand, and were not created strictly for peer review, they were discoverable.

---

232 *Hlall v. Lundman, Scott et al.,* Greene County (MO) County Court, case o. I 92CC2297.

9. HEALTH CARE IN THE REPUBLIC OF SERBIA

According to the structure of the legal system, the Republic of Serbia belongs to the group of countries of the continental legal system, which means that the legal norms are codified into corresponding regulations which regulate all areas of social life. The Constitution of the Republic of Serbia from 2006,[233] being the highest and essential legal act, builds from the basic principle that the legal order is unique and envisages the hierarchy of international regulations and regulations defined by the internal law in accordance with the principle of constitutionality and legality.[234] Article 68 of the Constitution of the Republic of Serbia stipulates that everybody has a right to the protection of his or her physical and mental health. This concerns the inalienable right of each citizen of the Republic of Serbia to have his or her physical and mental health protected in accordance with the law, while the law prescribes unconditional health care of certain vulnerable social categories (children, pregnant women, women who have just given birth, single parents with children up to seven years of aged and elderly persons), whose health care is provided from the public income unless they can claim the right to this kind of care other grounds.[235]

Health care in the Republic of Serbia is regulated by the Law on Health Care (hereinafter: LHC). This act defines health care as an organized and comprehensive activity of the society the aim of which is achieving the highest level of maintaining the health of citizens and the family, and it comprises the implementation of measures for maintaining and improving citizens' health, preventing, suppressing and early detection of illnesses, injuries and other health disorders, and timely and efficient treatments and rehabilitation.[236]

---

233 The Constitution of the Republic of Serbia, *The Official Gazelle of the Republic of Serbia No. 98/2006,*
234 Ayala, A., et al., *Ljudska prava u zdravstvenoj zastiti:* prirucnik za prakticare, Medicinski fakultet Univerziteta u Beogradu, 2015., p.203.
235 Pavlovic., B., Markovic, I., Cetkovic, P. *Pravo na zdravstvenu zastiti kroz prizmu lekarske greske,* Iustitia, Casopis udruzenja sudijskih i tuzilackih pomocnika Srbije, br. 1/2016, p.18-21.
236 Article 2 of the Law on Health Care, *"the Official Gazelle oft he Republic of Serbia",* No.25/2019.

In line with the LHC, each citizen of the Republic of Serbia and another persons with temporary or permanent residence in the territory of the Republic of Serbia is entitled to health care as well as a person in transit through the Republic of Serbia, who is entitled to urgent medical care. The provision of health care of the population is based on the principles of accessibility, fairness, comprehensiveness, continuity, constant improvement of health care quality and efficiency.[237]

The participants in health care in the Republic of Serbia, in line with the LHC, are as follows:[238] health care providers,[239] health insurance organizations, citizens, the family, employers, educational and other institutions, humanitarian, religious, sports and other organizations, associations, local government units, autonomous provinces and the Republic of Serbia.

Health care work is defined by the Law as work which ensures the health care of citizens and which is carried out through the health care system. Health care measures and activities must be based on scientific evidence, safe, effective and efficient, in line with the scientific standards, adopted guidebooks on good practices, protocols on medical treatment and principles of professional ethics.[240]

The Health care system in the Republic of Serbia is composed of medical institutions, higher-education institutions which run accredited study programs for acquiring proper knowledge and skills for carrying out health care work (hereinafter: higher-education medical institutions) and other legal entities which are foreseen by law a special law to carry out health care work additionally, private practice, health care workers and associates as well as the health care organization and financing.[241] The Republic

237 Paripovic, V., Rajakovic, D. Sistem zdravstvene zastite II Republici Srbiji, Iustitia, Casopis udruzenja sudijskih i tuzilackih pomocnika Srbije, br. 1/2016, str.29-30.
238 Article 4 of the Law on Health Care, "the Official Gazelle ofIl1e Republic of Serbia", No.25/2019.
239 Health care providers are as follows: l) state and private health-service institutions; 2) higher education medical institutions and other legal entities which are also foreseen to carry out health care work by virtue of a special Jaw (hereinafter: other legal entities); 3) private practice; 4) medical workers who carry out health care work in compliance with the Jaw; 5) other higher-education institutions, i.e. scientific-educational and scientific in titutions, accompanied by the opinion of the Ministry, in compliance with the Jaw. (Article 27 of the Law on Heath Care, „the Official Gazelle of the Republic of Serbia", o. 25/20 I 9.)
240 Article 5 of the Law on Health Care, "the Official Gazelle of the Republic of Serbia", No.25/2019.
241 Ibid. Article 6.

provides the means for taking social care for health at the level of the Republic, which are composed of measures of economic and social policies by which the conditions for the implementation of health care with a view preserving and improving the health of people are established as well well as of measures by which the functioning and the development of health care system are harmonized. The Law prescribes that the social care for the health of citizens is exercised at the level of the Republic, autonomous provinces, municipalities, i.e. towns, employers and individuals.[242]

In accordance with the LHC, a health-service institutions may be established from the state or privately owned funds. A state healthÂservice institution is founded by the Republic of Serbia, an autonomous province or a local governments unit, whereas a privately owned health-service institution is founded by a legal or natural person under the conditions stipulated by law. A health-service institution may be established as: a health center, polyclinic health care facility; a pharmacy facility; a hospital (general or special); a medical center; an institution; a public health institution; a clinic; an institute; a clinical hospital center; a university clinical center; a military medical institution or a sanitary institution or a unit in the Serbian Armed Forces, in line with a special law. The regulations governing the legal status of business organizations are applied accordingly to the authorities of a privately owned health-service institution, status changes, changes of the legal forms and closure. A health-service institution may also be established in line with the regulations governing public and private partnerships, unless it is regulated otherwise by this Law.[243]

In accordance with the LHC, a health-service institution may be founded and provide health care if it meets the prescribed conditions as regards the personnel (the prescribed type and the number of health care workers, i.e. medical associates with relevant university or high school education, who have passed the professional exam, who possess the relevant license for independent work which is issued by the competent chamber for carrying out certain work, who have specialized in a relevant area or have a relevant scientific or research title and who are employed on a permanent basis); the

---

242 Ibid. Article 8.
243 Ibid. Article 28.

207

equipment (prescribed diagnostic, therapeutic and other equipment for safe and modem provision of health care which the health-service institution has been established for); the space (prescribed rooms for the reception and accommodation of patients, for diagnostic, therapeutic and rehabilitative procedures, medical care as well as for storing medications and medical devices) and the availability of the appropriate type and quantity of medications and medical devices.

The health care work in the Republic of Serbia is carried out on three levels:

- On the primary level, health care comprises the protection and improvement of health, prevention and early detection of illnesses, treatments and rehabilitation, preventative health care, health care education and counseling, urgent medical assistance, pharmaceutical health protection etc. This form of health care is provided within a well developed network of health centers (at a municipal level) or by an individual doctor (in private practice). These are the institutions which the citizens may visit without a referral and where the citizens, as a rule, meet doctors for the first time. The team of selected doctors, which is composed of a general practitioner, a gynecologist, a pediatrician and a dentist constitute the basis of the primary health care organization. Apart from that, specialist and consultative work may also be conducted on the primary level.

- On the secondary level, health care is provided by specialist services (so called general specialist services), as a rule, in general or special hospitals, which usually represents the continuation of diagnostic, therapeutic or rehabilitative procedures which are, as a rule, initiated on the primary level. This level of care includes specialist and consultative and hospital health care which is provided by a (general or special) hospital. If a health center is unable to provide a required specialist health care, a doctor will refer a patient to the secondary level (a hospital). In hospitals in Serbia each patient will be provided with health care he or she requires: outpatient treatment (an examination by a specialist at a polyclinic) or inpatient treatment, i.e. lying in that hospital. Patients are referred to a hospital when their medical problem exceeds the technical conditions of a health center or the expert opinion of a higher level is required. [244]

---

244 Vodic kroz sisrem zdrovsrvene zasrire, available at: https://www.dzblace.org.rs/wpÂcontent/uploads/2014/04/VODIC-KROZ-SISTEM-ZDRA VSTVE E-ZASTITE.pdf.

- On the tertiary level, health care is provided by a clinic, an institute, a clinical hospital center and a clinical center. This level includes provision of the most complex forms of health care and specialist and consultative and hospital health care as well as scientific, research and educational work, and it represent a highly specialized or subspecialized level of health care. When a health problem exceeds the technical conditions of a hospital or an expert opinion of the highest level of health care is required, a patient is referred to a clinical center or one of the clinics, i.e. to an institute or a clinical hospital center. That is the tertiary and the ultimate level m the health care system in Serbia.[245]

Apart from the aforementioned, there are other health care facilities in the health care system, such as:[246] pharmacies, public health institutes, blood transfusion institutes and various institutes which may be on both the primary and the tertiary level in terms of administrative organization. Public health institutes are established for the territory of a district and they are in charge of public health activities on all three levels of administrative organization of the health care system in Serbia (Chart 1).[247]

---

245 Ibidem
246 For more information please see: Articles 74 - 90 of the Law on Health Care, "the Official Gazette of the Republic of Serbia", No.. 25/2019.
247 Ayala, A., i dr. op. cit.,pp.205.

Chart 1. Organizational structure of the health care system in Serbia

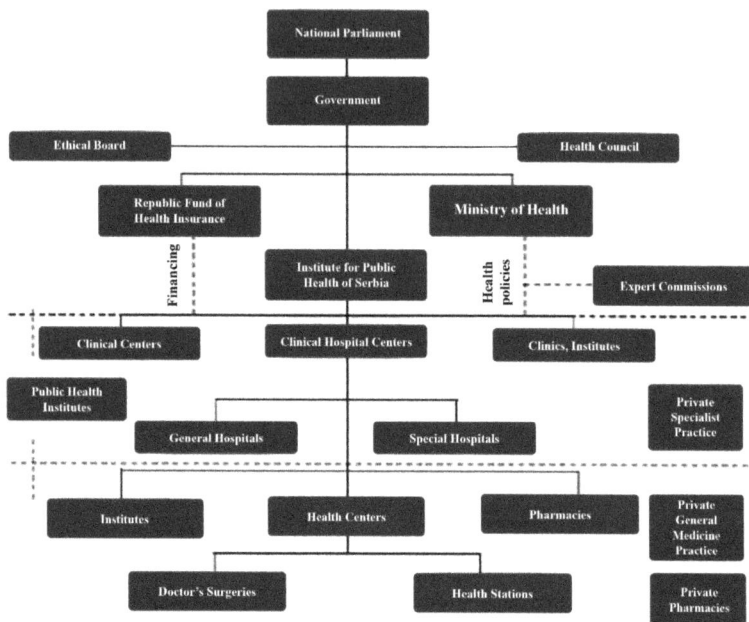

Source: Compilation from the Law on Health Care[248]

According to the way of financing, ownership, organization and health care system management, Serbia opts for the Bismarck Model. That means that the health care system is primarily financed from the mandatory health insurance contributions, which are paid by employees and their employers as well as other citizens who receive income (the founders of business enterprises, independent entrepreneurs, retired persons, agriculturalists). Contributions are collected and managed by the Republic Fund for Health Insurance. The health care system is additionally financed from other sources, public and private ones. In the public sources payments from the budget predominate, while the private sources are provided by the users of health services by direct payment for the services rendered, through voluntary health insurance, by a co-payment etc. In terms of obligatoriness, health insurance in Serbia may be compulsory and voluntary.[249]

---

248 Ibid., p. 206.
249 Ibid., p. 205-206.

In line with the LHC, health care may also be provided by other forms of health care services if they meet the conditions for a certain type of a health care institution, such as the medical faculties, social protection institutions, penitentiaries etc. Private practice may be founded by an unemployed health care worker who has passed the professional examination or a retired health care worker.

Private practice may be established as: a doctor's office, a dental office, a polyclinic, a laboratory, private practice pharmacy, a medical clinic and a dental technique laboratory. The founder of private practice has the status of a self-employed entrepreneur and he or she can found only one form of private practice. A health care worker may found private practice if he or she meets the conditions prescribed by the LHC, such as general medical fitness, possession of a relevant medical university degree or medical high school diploma, professional exam pass, entry in the directory of the competent chamber, work license etc. Private practice may also be established and provide health care if it meets the prescribed conditions in terms of personnel, equipment, space and the availability of the required type and quantity of medications and medical devices. Private practice may provide health care if the Ministry confirms by virtue of a decision that the prescribed conditions for providing health are fulfilled. Private practice may only engage in the health care activities defined by the decision on the fulfillment of the prescribed conditions for carrying our health care activities issued by the Ministry.[250]

Private practice is entered in the register of the Business Registers Agency (BRA) on the basis of the decision on the fulfillment of the prescribed conditions for providing health care,[251] in accordance with the law. Health care work defined by the decision issued by the Ministry of Health is entered in the register of the BRA. The register of health-services institutions and the Unique Records of Health Care Entities are kept by the BRA as entrusted work. Public and privately owned health-service institutions are entered into the Register in line with the law. The Register of health-service institutions is an electronic, central and public data base on registered health-service institutions which provide health care on the basis of the decision on the fulfillment

---

250 Article 40 of the Law on Health Care, "the Official Gazelle of the Republic of Serbia", No.25/2019.
251 Health-service institution foundation act is registered and published on the website of the Business Register Agency (BRA).

of the prescribed conditions for providing health care issued by a health inspector or a pharmaceutical inspector in accordance with the law. The unique records comprise complied data on health-service institutions and private practice in the territory of the Republic of Serbia. A health-service institution and private practice are entered in the register of the Business Register Agency when they start working.[252]

The supervision of the work of a health-service institution, other legal entities and private practice, as defined by the LHC, is done as the supervision of the enforcement of his law, regulations adopted for the implementation of this law as well as other regulations which govern the provision of health care and the right of patients, i.e. as inspection supervision. The work of a health-service institution, other legal entities or private practice is supervised by the Ministry through a health inspector, excluding the supervision over the work a pharmaceutical institution, a health center pharmacy as the organizational entity of another health-service institution, hospital pharmacy and the supervision over pharmaceutical activity, which is conducted through a pharmaceutical inspector in line with the law. The work of a health-service institution, other legal entities or private practice pursuant to Article 241, paragraph 1, of the LHC, which carry out health care work in the area of biomedicine is supervised m accordance with the regulations which govern biomedicine.[253]

Following the entry into the relevant Register, each health-service institution and private practice is obliged to maintain prescribed medical documentation [254] and to provide individual and collective reports to the competent public health institute by the prescribed deadline. Moreover, it should be mentioned that a health-service institution, private practice and other legal entities are obliged to keep medical documentation and records for the prescribed period of time. As it has already been mentioned, the work of a health-service institution, other legal entities and private practice are supervised, i.e. inspected by the Ministry of Health through a health inspector employed with the Health Inspection.

---

252 Article 46 of the Law on Health Care, "the Official Gazelle of the Republic of Serbia", No.25/2019.
253 Ibid, Article 241.
254 Medical documentation means an original or reproduced document taken into work or drafted within work of health-services institutions, private practice or other legal entities, while the medical records mean a document which contains noticed, measurable and repeatable result obtained during the examination of a patient as well as laboratory and diagnostic tests, evaluations or diagnostic formulations (Law on Medical Documentation and Records in Health Care, „the Official Gazelle of the Republic of Serbia", No. 123/2014, 106/2015, 105/2017 i 25/2019- other law),

The basic rights of patients are[255]: the right to the accessibility of health care, the right to information, the right to preventative measures, the right to quality, the right to the quality of the provided health care, the right to the safety of a patient, the right to being informed, the right to free choice, the right to the second expert opinion, the right to privacy and confidentiality, the right to consent, the right to the insight into the medical records, the right to the confidentiality of the data on the patient's health condition, the right to the relief of suffering and pain, the right to the respect for the patient's time and the right to an objection and the right to the damages.[256]

According to the LHC, the new health care technology means the medical technology that is introduced to the Republic of Serbia for the first time, i.e. at the certain level of health care. A health-service institution and private practice, a manufacturer, i.e. the holder of the license for a medical device submit the request for the issuance of a license for the use of new health care technology to the Ministry of Health. Based on the prior opinion given on the assessment of health care technology, the Minister issues a license for new health care technology by virtue of a decision, which contains the conditions for the application of new health care technology, the level of assessed risk from harmful effects on the life ans health of a patient, i.e. the population, as well as the level of health care at which it is applied. New health care technology may be applied in the health care system at the level of health care for which the license for use has been issued.[257]

---

255 The term patient denotes a person, i.e. an insured person as defined by the Law on Health Insurance, either ill or healthy, who seeks or is provided with a health service for maintaining or improving health, prevention, suppression or early detection of an illness, injury or other health disorder and timely and efficient treatment and rehabilitation (Article 2 of the Law on Patient Rights, *"the Official Gazelle of the Republic of Serbia"*, No. 45/2013 i 25/2019 - other laws)
256 Ibid, Article 6 - 3 I.
257 Article 51 of the Law on Health Care, *"the Official Gazelle of1he Republic of Serbia"* No. 25/2019

The expert methodological instructions for employing the methods of "anti-aging" medicine[258] define precise conditions, ways and procedures of using "anti-aging" medicine methods in a health-service institution or private practice and conditions which have to be fulfilled by the continuing education program educators as well as other significant matters through which the conditions for obtaining licenses for "anti-aging" medicine are fulfilled. Up to that period, this area was not adequately legally regulated and untimely action of the health care competent authorities towards legally defining this form of health care technology has led to frequent commissions of criminal offenses against the human health, accompanied by serious consequences such as grave bodily injury or grave damage to the health of patients subjected to this medical procedures.

In accordance with the mentioned instructions, the aesthetic "anti-aging" medicine procedures are: skin, subcutaneous tissue and mucous membrane volume replacement with the aim of removing signs of aging (dermal fillers injecting), botulinum toxin application - wrinkle correction, minimally invasive face lifting techniques - thread lifting, regenerative medicine - application with the removal of signs of aging; PRP technique of injecting in aesthetic medicine - the removal of the signs of aging on the facial and body skin and other similar techniques, mesotherapy - application in aesthetic medicine and for treatment, chemical peeling, collagen induction therapy, carboxytherapy, electromagnetic radiation: non-ablative fractional rejuvenation of the skin surface, treatments with the intensive pulsed lights, excluding the area around eyes, photo-dynamic therapy, radio frequency treatment for skin straightening, infrared light devices and other devices for skin straightening treatment, lasers, infrared light treatments, radio frequency therapy, intensive pulsed light treatments and other sources of equivalent power which is applied to the area around eyes, high frequency, radio frequency and other treatments by means of devices based on

---

258 „Anti-aging" medicine represents the form of new health care technology which involves methods and procedures of the prevention, diagnostics, treatments and rehabilitation of changes occurring as a consequence of aging, i.e. methods the application of which has a beneficial effect on health and physical appearance. The mentioned methods as a new form of health care technologies are not specifically included in the study courses of the academic studies of medicine and dentistry, but they are directly linked to certain acquired knowledge and skills in the mentioned scientific areas. *The Expert Methodological Instuctions for Employing the Mei hods of "Anti-aging" Medicine* o. 500-01-1246/2018-02 of 19.09.2018, p. 1-2.

energy the temperature of which rises to above 42 °c, LED light (light emitting diodes) treatments and focused ultrasound.[259]

The mentioned "anti-aging" medical procedures may be performed exclusively in health-service institutions and private practice founded as a general or specialist doctor's office, dental office or a polyclinic, which have been issued with the license for a certain "anti-aging" medicine procedure by virtue of the decision made by the minister of health in order to be able to perform those medical procedures. The performance of the mentioned "anti-aging" medicine procedures is not allowed in beauty and other salons nor is it allowed in any other space which is not a health-service institution of the mentioned private practice, regardless of the fact whether the service is provided by a doctor or another health care worker. "Anti-aging" medicine medical procedures which are performed in health-service institutions or private practice registered for surgical branches of medicine, or dental medicine, and which are not registered for inpatient treatment, are performed in health-service institutions and private practice as new health care technology procedures. These medical procedures may be performed with the supply of both appropriate kinds and quantities of medications and medical devices registered by the Agency for medications and Medical Devices. A founder of private practice is obliged to place the photocopy of the license for the introduction of new health care technologies in "anti-aging" medicine issued by the Ministry of Health on a noticeboard on the premises of private practice in addition to the data posted in line with the regulation stipulating precise requirements for providing health care in health-service institutions and other forms of health care services.[260]

---

259 *Strucno melodolosko uputstvo za obavljanje meloda „Anliage" medicine* No. 500-01-1246/2018-02 of 19.09.2018, p. 2-3. Pravilnik o blizim uslovima i nacinu vrsenja procene zdravstvenih tehnologija, „Sluzbeni glasnik RS", No. 97/20)
260 Ibid., p. I - 2.

215

The Law on Health Care Workers' Chambers[261] lays down the obligation that the membership of a chamber (the Serbian Medical Chamber, the Serbian Dental Chamber, the Pharmaceutical Chamber of Serbia, the Serbian Chamber of Biochemists, the Chamber of Nurses and Health Care Technicians of Serbia) is mandatory for all doctors of medicine, dentists, graduate pharmacists, graduate pharmacists of medical biochemistry, graduate specialist pharmacists of medical biochemistry and specialist doctors of medicine of clinical biochemistry, nurses and health care technicians, which provide health care by profession in health-service institutions and other forms of health care services in the Republic of Serbia.[262] The mentioned chambers have registers, i.e. data bases of doctors with a valid license and a work permit, where the information on whether a certain doctor has a work license or works without a license may be quickly retrieved by accessing the websites of the chambers.

Registration of a health-service institution/private practice or another legal entity in the official Register with the Business Register Agency (BRA) offers the possibility of obtaining important information on health care providers (date of foundation and entry in the Register, line of work, data on the head office, responsible person, founders, the amount of capital, bank accounts numbers, published documents - on the status etc.) by searching the Register on the internet. Health care providers such as health-service institutions, private practice and other legal entities which provide health care are obliged to record their financial transactions via current accounts, where the Unique Register of Accounts of the National Bank of Serbia may serve as a source as to whether they record their financial transactions effect via current accounts. The financial transactions of the legal entities founded by the Republic of Serbia are carried out via the accounts, and the records on that are kept by the Treasury Administration of the Republic of Serbia.

The professional status of a doctor or another health care worker as regards taking decisions on sensitive issues of human health and life entails special personal responsibility and duty of a doctor to provide adequate health service in accordance with the Code of Medical Ethics of the Serbian Medical Chamber. 263

---

261 The Law on Health Care Workers' Chambers, *"the Official Gazelle of the Republic of Serbia",* No. 107/2005, 99/2010 i 70/2017-Constitution Court Decision.
262 Ibid., Article 4.
263 *"The Official Gazelle of the Republic of Serbia",* No. 104/2016.

10. CRIMINAL ACTS IN THE AREA OF TREATMENTS AND PROVISION OF OTHER MEDICAL SERVICES

DEFINITIONS AND THE BASIC ELEMENTS OF CRIMINAL ACTS

When speaking of criminal acts, it is necessary to start from their defining. There is no unique definition which describes them in a universal or comprehensive way nor are there definite and invariable rules for their defining as it concerns an extremely complex and dynamic negative social phenomenon. We encounter a multitude of definitions which describe a criminal act in literature and practice.

Crime - (*lat. crimen* - felony) is a negative social phenomenon which represents a set of activities of one or more persons which are contrary to legal regulations and standards of conduct, the disregard and violation of which involves a relevant sanction, the type and severity of which depends on the level of social risk posed by the acts committed. A criminal act is the result of human behaviour and thus it can be defined as human conduct which has a harmful effect on the society, which responds to it by applying a criminal sanction to the one who has committed that act. Criminal behaviour or deliberate misleading of an individual, a group or an organization is based upon the intention to achieve an aim, i.e. to satisfy a certain personal need in a dishonest and irregular way. The number of instances and the content of punishable acts has changed with the development of the society and culture. Criminality is not static and fixedly determined, it changes all the time.[264]

---

[264] According to the majority of authors, those types of conduct which are incriminated in the valid criminal legislation as criminal offenses constitute criminality. There is also a wider legal definition within the legal determining of the term criminality according to which the term criminality extends to all punishable acts in a certain legal system. Criminality denotes each instance of illegal conduct (doing or omission to do) for which a competent authorities may impose a sanction in accordance with the valid regulation of a certain country. For n1ore details, please see: NikoliC-RistanoviC, V., Konstantinovic-Vilic, S. *Kriminologija*, „Prometcj", Beograd, 2018., p.23.

Criminal acts are the subject of constant interest of scientists and practitioners for being widespread and for social risk. This concerns the acts which arouse the attention of expert and general public for difference in commission, the volume and the intensity of ensuing consequences, i.e. the activities which criminologists, criminal-law experts, lawyers, forensic accountants, psychologists, psychiatrists, forensic medicine experts, sociologists and other professionals deal with theoretically and in practice. They are as old as the human kind, but they have evolved throughout the development of the society. The comprise a wide range of manifestations which are characterized by deliberate deception or misrepresentation, which are done with the aim of making illegal gain for an individual or an organization, while their perpetrator may be outside or within that organization.[265]

Different terms for denoting certain forms and manners of commission of criminal acts are used in theory and practice, such as: *"fraud", 'fraudulent act, , "illegal activity/act", "malfeasance", "manipulation", "deception", "theft", "misuse", "embezzlement", "irregularity", "negligence", "misrepresentation", "concealment", "cheating"* etc. These key words indicate that relates to the activities which are undertaken, i.e. committed by an individual, an employee or a manager in an organization with the aim of making illegal financial gain or gaining advantage, which would not have happened unless these activities were undertaken.

The right to professional practice of medicine is directly linked to the duty to provide health care to those who seek it, considering the fact that the provision of health services is an important determinant of the profession in line with the provisions of the LHC.[266]

In medical profession, as it is the case with all professions and activities, there are individuals/groups who work contrary to the nterests of their colleagues as well as the society on the whole. Fraudulent activities in health care represent a huge problem in all countries of the world, which, as a negative phenomenon, significantly deplete the resources of health-service institutions, companies, state health care programs, thus reducing the supplies for the treatment of seriously ill patients.

---

265 Cvetkovic D. Banovic, B. *Upravljanje rizicima od prevara sa aspeka forenzickog racunovodstva*, Zbornik radova naucne konferencije: Finansijski kriminalitet i korupcija, Instin,t za uporedno pravo, Institut za kriminoloska i socioloska istrazivanja, Beograd, Vrsac, 2019., p. 243-258.
266 The Law on Health Care „*the Official Gazelle of the Republic of Serbia*" No.25/2019.

Although a very small number of participants in health care engages in fraudulent activities, the consequences affect all participants. This, for instance, leads to the reduction/curtailing of public revenue of the social community, payment of a higher insurance policy for employees by their employers, i.e. higher costs of health care, which can result in limited availability of services provided by health care institutions.

According to the definition of the *Centers for Medicare & Medicaid Services (CMS)*,[267] a fraud in health care is deliberate deception or misrepresentation of facts or actions which an individual executes within health care system and which he or she knows or should know to be false or does not believe to be true, but with the help of which that individual or another person may have unlawful benefit. The US Health Insurance Portability and Accountability Acts defines a fraud in health care as knowing or willful execution or an attempt at execution of actions with the aim of embezzlement of any health care benefit program by means of false claims, representations or promises of money or property which are owned by any health care benefit program. In Chapter 18 of the US Code, health care fraud is defined as a criminal act, namely as knowing and willful execution of actions or their fabrication with a view to defrauding any health health care benefit program or with the aim of making (by false pretenses or promises) any kind of financial gain or acquiring (im)material assets owned by or under the control of any health care benefit program."[268] The criminal acts, i.e. health care fraud may also be defined as activities which are not in accordance with good medical and business practice.

267 Medicare and Medicaid programs in the US are equivalent to many programs sponsored by the governments of other, primarily well developed countries. Regardless of the state in question, the existence of the continuum of health care and the roles in it are the same. All health care system have patients, health care providers, administrative services, sponsors for the implementation of health care payment plans (usually via the countries' government programs or though private health insurance) and additional sellers of health services, equipment or material. For more information please see: ikolovski, S., *Prevarne radnje u zdravstvu i specificnosti njihovog identijikovanja*, grupa autora, Forenzicko racunovodstvo, istrazne radnje, ljudski faktor i primenjeni ala ti, p. 517-548, the Faculty of Organized Sciences, Belgrade, 2021
268 Health Insurance Portability and Accountability Act 1996 (18 U.S.C., ch. 63, sec.1347.
Opsimije: ikolovski, S., (2021). „*Prevame radnje u zdravstvu i specificnosri njihovog idemifikovanja*", gmpa autora, Forenzicko racunovodstvo, istrazne radnje, ljudski faktor i primenjeni alati, p. 517-548, the Faculty of Organized Sciences, Belgrade

Fraudulent acts bear in themselves an element of concealment and employee collusion. Controlling and managing structures should have systematic knowledge of the existence of specifically designed control procedures for countering manipulations.[269] Although there are several definitions of criminal acts in the context of health care, all definitions have two common characteristics: 1. incorrect statements, i.e. making false statements or claims, concealing (obscuring) facts related to the provision of medical services and misrepresentation of facts and, based on that, 2. causing damage to another person, a group, an organization, a country or the community on the whole.[270]

The term "health care fraud" refers to a wide range of deviant behaviours which occur within the activity of providing and trade in medical services. In addition to different kinds, there are also different levels of fraud, which private and state subjects are related to and the response to which can be various sanctions. Apart from filing a criminal charge or a claim for damages in legal proceedings, citizens also have several more methods for the protection and claiming their rights at their disposal. The Law on the Protection of Patients' Right stipulates the fundamental right of a patient to objection, if he or she thinks that he or she has been deprived of health care in a health service institution or any other legal entity which provides medical services or that he or she has had that right denied by an act committed by a medical worker or associate.[271] These legal remedies and sanctions may be criminal, civil or administrative. Appropriate sanctions for a certain case depend on its concrete facts. In many situations, the efficient access to clinical records via interoperable electronic health records can be a powerful tool for tackling potentially fraudulent behaviour.[272]

---

269 Petkovic, A., Cvetkovic, D. *Interne kontrole protiv kriminalnih radnji u fimkciji pouzdanog finansijskog izvesravanja.* Revizor, Belgrade, 2018., 21(82), p. 33-44.
270 Foundation of Research and Education American Health Information Management Association. Report on the Use of Health Infonnation Technology to Enhance and Expand Health Care Anti-Fraud Activities. Chicago, IL; 2005.
271 Ayala, A., i dr. op. cit., p.392.
272 ikolovski, S. op. cit., p. 517-548.

Fraud in health care is widely spread and it has no limits. The Institute for Medicine of National Academies estimates that the US citizens suffer the damage of 7 5 US dollars at the expense of fraudulent acts in health care annually.[273] The US Department of Justice charged 2.5 billions of US dollars via settlements and verdicts for fraudulent acts and false claim in the health care system in 2016. The American Government and the Department of Justice are very creative in developing legal theories for the fight against fraud and misuse in health care. Thus, the competences of the US Government extended to the fight against fraud and misuse by virtue of the Patient Protection and Affordable Care Act from 2010 and Health Care and Education Reconciliation Act (known as Health Care Reform Act).[274]

The group of authors describe the triangle of a criminal act which explains why criminal acts occur. Namely, the research and the analysis of risk elements of criminal behaviour, by which the assets are appropriated illegally by an individual or a group, has led to three crucial factors for unlawful activities in disposing of another person's property. These factors are typically called "the triangle for the occurrence of a criminal act",[275] as they represent the associated conditions that one is induced and decides to commit such an act. There are three common factors which characterize a criminal act, so called fraud triangle, which contains three basic elements :[276]

pressure/motive/need or incentive, which is defined as motivation or as a need that cannot be shared with others;

Opportunities and knowledge, i.e. the possibility of committing a criminal act without being discovered;

Justifying attitude/rationalization, i.e. an excuse, which is based on the personal attitude on ethics.

---

273 http://www.nationalacademies.org/hmd/Reports/20 12/Best-Care-at-Lower-Cost-The-Path-to-Continuously-Learn ing-Health-Care-in-A merica .aspx.
274 ikolovski, S., op.cit, p. 517-548.
275 Fraud triangle was developed by Donald R. Cressey (1950.), and that is the most traditional theory for discovering fraud (Saluja, S., A. Aggarwal & A. Mittal *Undersranding the fraud theories and advancing wilh inregrily model,* Journal of Financial Crime, 2021, ahead-of-print No. ahead-of-print. https://doi. org/ l0.1108/JFC-07-2021-0163.).
276 Cvetkovic 0., MiCoviC D., To1niC, M. Forensic accounting and criminal work in commercial sceilies, Zbomik radova Medunarodnog naucnog skupa ,Dani Arcibalda Rajsa", Tom I, Kriminalisticko-policijska akademija, Beograd, 2018., p. 125 -136.

Picture I. Fraud triangle (Skalak, et.al., remodelled)[277]

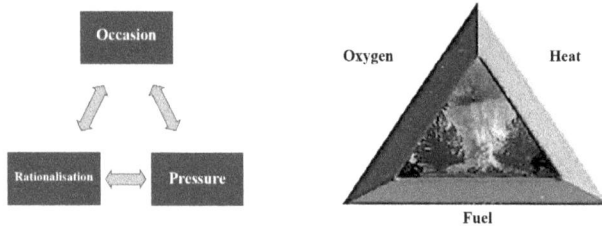

a) Each kind of pressure to tum to an action for committing fraud may be subsumed under the term motive. These motives may be diverse: psychological motives, egocentric, ideological, economic etc. (e.g. a personal financial problem).

b) Circumstances lead to the possibility of the management or an employee committing fraud. The observed possibility for committing a certain form of a fraudulent act, for concealing it or for avoiding punishment is another element in the fraud triangle. There are at list six main factors within this element which strengthen the possibility of individuals committing a criminal act and they are as follows:[278]

Lack or evasion of controls which prevent or detect criminal acts

Inability to assess the quality of the work done

Failure to punish a perpetrator of a criminal act

Lack of access to information

Ignorance, apathy and incapacity

Lack of revision track

---

277 Skalak, Golden, Clyton & Pill. *A Guide to Forensic Accounting Investigarion,* New York, John Wiley and Sons Inc., 2011.
278 Albrecht, W. Steven., Albrecht, Chad. *Fraud Examination&Prevention,Thomson-South-Western,* Ohio, 2004., p. 26.

c) Pretext for committing unlawful acts is the third and the last motivating factor which induces a person to engage in commission of various forms of fraud. Persons who commit fraud simply do not admit that they have committed it. They justify themselves by claiming that they are not doing anything bad or different from the others. They believe that if conditions, according to them, are pointless or they do not like them, they can "evade" them. They lie to themselves that it is just "this time". This cannot be stopped easily and it results in falling deeper into fraud. The psychological complexity of an employee can often be the cause; certain employees are more oriented to fraud considering the fact that they do not have stable motivation. In fraud, the most frequent attitude could be the following:[279] "My needs are greater then those of other people, "I only borrow money - I am returning them", "No person suffered damage", "The company is too big to feel it", "Everybody does that", "I deserve more for my work", „Nobody will be hurt", , "This was done with good intentions.", "We will take care of the papers as soon as we are out of financial difficulties" etc.

Regardless of the participants in fraudulent acts, one of the key elements of health care fraud (or any other kind of fraud, regardless of the area in which it occurs) is the fact that individuals who commit these acts display partial or absolute absence of conscience. Many world analysts in this area link the commission of such fraudulent acts to antisocial personality disorder which has prevalence of over 4%, which represents around 300 million people across the world with perfect psychological profile for the commission of fraud. This condition is discussed for the fact that there are precisely established criteria which are used for making the diagnosis. Those criteria for antisocial personality disorder, at least three of which must be present to reach the diagnosis, are as follows: failure to conform to the social norms, deceitfulness and tendency to manipulation, impulsiveness and lack of success in advance planning, irritability and aggressiveness, reckless disregard for personal safety and safety of others, consistent irresponsibility and lack of remorse after harming, maltreating or stealing the property of another person.[280]

279 Cvetkovic O., Micovic O., Tomic, M. op. cit., str. 125 -136.
280 Ikolovski, S. *Prevara i zloupotreba u zdravsrvenom sistemu,* grupa autora, Prevamo finansijsko izvestavanje: metode, snidije slucaja I istrage, p. 21-63, Preduzece za reviziju, racunovodstvene, finansijske i konsalting usluge „Moodys standards" d.o.o. Beograd, 2022.

Another clear sign is direct denial of an event, despite the existence of irrefutable evidence. Apart from that, it often happens that the statements of the accused of fraud do not correspond to known and confirmed events. There is frequently a lack of any emotional response or, on the other hand, there is an inconsistent emotional reaction in comparison to established social norms, not only in cases of fraud investigation, but also in conversations about other life situations of the accused in which a certain emotional reaction is physiological and expected. Another key indicator is the series of failures for the lack of planning and consistent irresponsibility in various spheres of life, and not only in planning the commission of fraudulent acts.[281]

The aforementioned elements are typical of each fraud, whether a fraudulent act in favour of an individual or in favour of organization is in question. Many authors compare the occurrence of a criminal act with the possibility of fire outbreak. According to them, "a fraudulent act resembles a fire in many ways. Three elements are required for a fire to break out: 1) oxygen, 2) fuel, 3) heat. Those three elements make "a fiery triangle" and when all three elements merge, a fire breaks out."[282]

Apart from that, some of the analyses suggest that it is necessary to add the fourth concept - *the ability of an individual (Fraud Diamond Theo,y FDT)* (Picture 2). The fact that somebody can or is induced to commit a theft does not necessarily mean that he or she is able to do it. For instance, if somebody does not understand how business transactions are recorded in accounting books (a register, a ledger,auxiliary books), it is logical to conclude that he or she would not be able to manipulate figures despite the inducement or an opportunity.[283]

---

281 Ibidem.
282 Albrecht, W. Steven., Albrecht , Chad., Fraud Examination&Prevention, Thomson-South-Western, Ohio, 2004, str. 20.
283 For more details please see: Knezevic, S. et al. „Razvoj kapacitela forenzickog racunovodstva" gmpa autora, Prevamo finansijsko izveslavanje: melode, studije slucaja i istrage, Preduzece za reviziju, racunovodstvene, finansijske i konsahing usluge „Moodys standards" d.o.o. Beograd, 2022., p.63-98.

Picture 2. Fraud Diamond

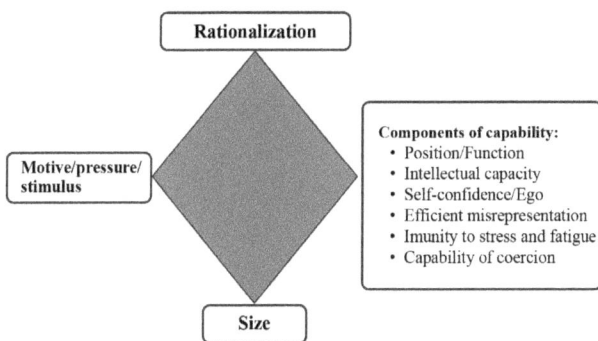

Source: Knezevic, S et al. *"Razvoj kapaciteta forenzickog racunovodstva"* grupa autora, Prevarno finansijsko izvestavanje: metode, studije slucaja i istrage, Preduzece za reviziJu, racunovodstvene, finansijske i konsalting usluge „Moodys standards" d.o.o. Beograd, 2022., p.63-98.

What follows from the aforesaid is that criminal acts/health care frauds are widely spread. Although a small percentage of participants in health care system commits these incriminating acts, the consequences affect all the participants. The basic elements detected in health care fraudulent acts are: the absence of conscience, failure to implement those segments of fraudulent acts which were not planned in detail or which were heedlessly performed by the perpetrators.

When the question as to why criminal acts occur is answered, factors which increase the risk from frauds should be identified, and risk factors are associated with three previous common factors which characterize a criminal act. It is extremely important to observe the main reason for committing frauds in an organization. Thus, the assessment of the risk from fraud and the establishment of adequate corrective and protective procedures for the future is easier. In many cases, professional investigators are required for examinations or other factors. Moreover, it is necessary to talk to lawyers as well. When a fraud is discovered, full investigation must follow. The investigation into fraud is conducted with a view to recovering the lost amount of money, dismissing or punishing the perpetrators, preventing its recommision and absolving the innocent persons of guilt. Investigations into frauds must provide evidence on the loss, dishonesty and enable the preparation for bringing a criminal charge.[284]

---

284 Cvetkovic O. Banovic, B. op. cit, p. 243-258.

Table 1: Evolution of typical criminal acts

1	Motivation/Pressure - need, greed, revenge
2	Possibility (lack in control) - access to resources, records, documents
	a. There is no revision hack or separation of duties
	b. There is no rotation of duties
	c. There is no function of internal revision
	d. There are no policies regarding control
	e. There is no code of ethics
	f. /
3	Excuses (formulation of intention) - justification that this act is a loan and not theft
4	Commission of the criminal act - certain criminal schemes: criminal acts, thefts, embezzlement etc.
5	Realization - theft of supplies, conversion of securities, cheques into cash
6	Concealment of the criminal act - altering of documents, destruction of records, forging
7	Warning signs - inconsistencies arc detected, there are assumptions, changes in behaviour pattern arc observed with the perpetrator (if scams can be tracked through business records,warning signs arc found in accounting books, and if they cannot be tracked in that way, then the warning sign is behaviour)
8	Revision commences - tips, internal control, accidental discovery, internal revision, identified and defined anomalies are used for criminal purposes
9	Investigation is launched - evidence is collected, loss of n1eans is confirmed and documented, third persons are examined, employees who have certain knowledge and suspects
10a	Taking measures - the perpetrator is identified - management does not want to resort to prosecution; insurance claim is submitted
10b	Taking measures - prosecution is recommended - prosecution is sought, civil suit, insurance claim is submitted
11	Court proceedings - presentation of facts and testifying

PERPETRATORS AND MANIFESTATIONS OF CRIMINAL ACTS IN TREATMENTS AND PROVISION OF OTHER MEDICAL SERVICES

Criminal acts in treatments and provision of medical services may be committed anywhere and by any person or a group. Namely, all participants in health care system are potential perpetrators of frauds. Thus, they can be committed by health care providers, on the one hand, and patients, on the other, as well as by other actors in the health care sector (insurance companies, companies which operate within pharmaceutical industry, medical equipment manufacturers as well as many other medical and non-medical participants who benefit from these acts). Therefore, the list of potential perpetrators comprise the service providers (employers and employees of health-service institutions); patients; individuals, domestic or foreign; employees who make false allegations about themselves or others; organized criminal groups involved in health care fraud; non/medical individuals who provide health service, but also create fraud patterns; retailers and suppliers who provide services within special health care system industries etc.

Health care fraud may placed under the category of frauds committed by service providers, services users (a patient or an insured person) and frauds committed by insurance institutions or payers of services. The most common type of a criminal act in health care involves a false statement, misrepresentation or deliberate omission of facts. A perpetrator of fraudulent acts may be a doctor or another individual provider of medical services, a hospital or another institutional health care provider, a clinical laboratory or another supplier, an employee of any participant in the health care system chain, an administrative organization, a user of medical service, an employee in an organization implementing a health plan or any other person within the health care system which may benefit from such acts. Thus, criminal acts may be committed by individuals, but also by groups of people or institutions. It rarely happens that the aim of perpetrators of criminal acts is to cause damage to only one of the insured persons or the state or the private sector exclusively. In the majority of cases, much larger number of persons insured with both private and public health care sector is damaged at the same time.[285]

---

285 ikolovski, S. op. cit., p. 21-63.

The data on the characteristics of the perpetrators of health care criminal acts are very scarce worldwide and that predominantly relates to the countries with low or middle level of development. The US has made the data on the characteristics of doctors involved in criminal acts within their health care systems widely available, so they are practically the only available data so that an insight into the current state of this subject matter would be gained to a certain extent. The total exclusion of doctors from the US public insurance funds increased by 20% on average annually in the period between 2007 and 2017, which resulted in the total rise of approximately 200% by the end of that ten-year period. The main causes of these increases are criminal acts. The exclusion of doctors which are related to unlawful prescribing of controlled substances had a smaller share in the total number of exclusions, which, especially in this category, increased by 21 % on average annually within the same time period.[286]

Table 2. Main aims of the commission of criminal acts in the health care system

Main aims of commission of frauds in the health care system
Search for money
Evasion of responsibility
Malicious causing of damage
Gaining competetive advantage
Gaining advantage in the field of research and on medical products market
Addiction
Theft of personal belongings
Theft of identity of an individual or an organization

Source: Nikolovski, S., *Prevara i zloupotreba u zdravstvenom sistemu*, grupa autora, Prevarno finansijsko izvestavanje: metode, studije slucaja i istrage, p. 21-63, Preduzece za reviziju, racunovodstvene, finansijske i konsalting usluge „Moodys standards" d.o.o. Belgrade, 2022.

---

286 *Ibid., p. 21-63.*

In the period between 2007 and 2017, 2,222 doctors (0,29%) were temporarily or permanently excluded from Medicare and other state programs of the US public insurance, mostly for unlawful prescribing of controlled substances or criminal acts. Statistically, the doctors who obtained degrees in medicine abroad, male doctors and doctors above 35 years of age were excluded from the health insurance programs significantly more frequently in comparison to other groups. The most often excluded doctors were specialists in family medicine, psychiatry, internal medicine, anesthesiology, surgeons, gynecologists and obstetricians, while it was most rarely the case with cardiologists and radiologists. The doctors bearing the title of doctors of osteopathic medicine, which is very popular in the US, the doctors who worked in rural areas and those who did not have additional academic positions at medical universities were also in greater risk of being excluded from public insurance funds for fraudulent acts.[287]

Damage inflicted to health care systems across the world as a result of criminal acts is enormous. The fact which is even more alarming is that the analysis of that damage does not exist in the majority of countries. Naturally, the United State have gone the furthest in this respect, as it is the case in the majority of other fields. In that country, twice as much money is expended on the implementation of health care in comparison to the greatest number of other developed countries. Nevertheless, the US national statistics in the health care system show increasingly bad picture.[288] According to the American Institute for Medicine, the damage caused to the US by fraud and misuse in 2019 amounted to 750 billion of dollars (28% of the total annual expenditure on health care), out of which fraud alone damaged the country in the amount of 75 billion dollars (3% the total expenditure on health care).[289] Other resources, including the Federal Bureau of Investigation (FBI), claim that the total damage inflicted to the US as a result of fraudulent charges in 2010 reached up to 260 billion dollars (10% of the total expenditure on health care).[290]

287 Chen, A., D. Blumenthal & A. Jena. *Characterislics of Physicians Excluded from US* Medicare and State Public Insurance Programs for Fraud, Health Crimes, or Unlawful Prescribing of Controlled Substances. JAMA Network Open , 1(8), el 85805. 2018, hllps://doi.org/10.100l/jamanetworkopen .2018.5805.
288 Hoffer, E. *The American Health Care Sysrem Is Broken.* Part 7: How Can We Fix It?. The American Journal of Medicine, 132(12), 1381-1385. hnps://doi.org/10.1016/j.amjmed. 2019.10.003.
289 Institute of Medicine. *Best Care at Lower Cost:* The Path to Continuously Leaming Health Care in America. Washington, DC: ational Academies Press, 2012 .
290 *Federal Bureau of Investigation.* Financial crimes report 2010-2011. https://www.fbi.gov/stats-services/publications/financial-crimes-report-2010-2011.

Criminal acts in health care represent a national epidemic in the US, which devastates public finances and government health care programs. Although the exact amount of damage for committed criminal acts in health care in the US cannot be established with certainty, as the majority of them is never discovered, it is estimated that it is around 3-10% of all health care costs, i.e. 68-226 billion of dollars annually.[291,292] Even the average value of these two estimated sums would be enough to cover health insurance of each uninsured US citizen.[293 294]

The costs of health system go up rapidly in most parts of the world. At global level, around 10% gross domestic product is spent on health care.[295] Unfortunately, all that money does not go to the right place, and consequently up to 10% of total costs in the health care system is spent as the result of committing frauds and misuse, which amounts to several billions of dollars annually.[296]

Health care is a dynamic market among the sellers, i.e. health services/resources providers and their users, and the system involves several groups of members. A patient is an individual who receives a medical service, whereas a health service provider is a physical or a legal entity who offers or provides a medical service. Insurance companies are the subjects which most usually make payments for services used and for used medications, equipment and material, and they can be private as well as state-owned, such as countries' governments programs. The most common type of health care fraud is a false statement, misrepresentation or omission of facts and it can be committed by individuals or groups of people and institutions. Those who suffer the consequences of fraudulent acts mainly comprise several insured persons or other persons simultaneously or even the entire public or private sector.

291 National Health Care Anti-Fraud Association (NHCAA "The problem of health care fraud") 2008, available at: www.nhcaa.org/resources/health-care-anti-fraud-resources/ the problem- of-health-care-fraud.aspx.
292 Federal Bureau of Investigation (FBI) 2009 Financial Crimes Report, available at: www.fbi.gov/stats-services/publications/financialcrimes-report-2009 (accessed on 8'" of April, 2012).
293 Ikolovski, S., op. cit.,p. 21-63.
294 Hadley, J. & J. Holahan, The cost of care for rhe uninsured: what do we spend, who pays, and what would full coverage add to medical spending?", 2004., available at: www.kff.org/uninsured/upload/the-cost-of-care-for-the-uninsured-what-do-we-spend-who-pays-andwhat-would-full-coverage-add-to-medical-spending.pdf.
295 Health Financing. World Health Organization. Available at: http://www.who.int/gho/health_financinglen/index.html.
296 Gee, J, M. Button, G. Brooks & P. Vincke, The financial cost of healthcare fraud. Portsmouth: University of Portsmouth, MacIntyre Hudson, Milton Keynes. Avai;able at: http://eprints.port.ac.uk/3987/l/The-Financial-Co t-of-Healthcare-Fraud-Final-(2). pdf.

What is necessary is that any actor in the chain of provision of medical services displays in his or her work deviant conduct which varies from the standard prescribed norms in such a way that damage is inflicted to another person (see picture - diagram of the continuum of fraudulent acts).[297]

Picture 3-diagram of the continuum of fraudlent acts[298]

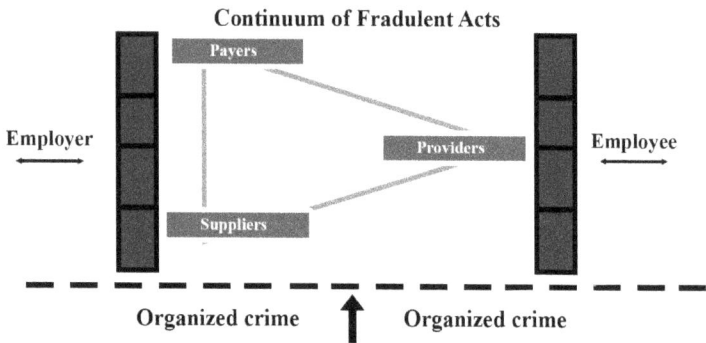

Continuum of Fradulent Acts

Payers

Employer

Providers

Employee

Suppliers

Organized crime   Organized crime

The most common manifestations of criminal acts in the area of health services provision and health care are as follows:[299]

Fraud by emergency medical services.

Charging services which are generally not charged.

Charging services which were not provided or the material which was not used.

Charging unnecessary services, examinations and tests.

Charging services provided by a medical worker although he or she was not present.

Corruption.

Double charging.

Fraud relating to the permanent equipment by a supplier.

Reports on false costs.

Presentation of incorrect dates of the provision of services. Presentation of incorrect locations of the provision of services.

False reporting of diagnoses or procedures.

---

297 Jbid., p. 517-548.
298 Ibid., p. 517-548.
299 Piper, C. *Healthcare fraud investigation guidebook*. Boca Raton, FL: Taylor & Francis Group, 2016.

Laboratory work fraud.

Misrepresentation of the patient's name.

Misrepresentation of the service provider's name.

Fraud in relation to medications which are issued on a prescription. Reporting and charging two or more services which should be reported under one code as one service.

Reporting a service which is more expensive that the one which was actually rendered and which is similar to it.

Reporting and charging a longer treatment although the time spent providing the service was much shorter.

Appropriation of patients' additional payments to insurance companies.

Apart from the aforementioned, manifestations of criminal acts in the area of provision of medical services and health care also include the following:

Provision of a medical service by an incompetent, unqualified person who misrepresents himself or herself as a medical expert;

Performing activities which are not in accordance with the health care provision standard;

Inadequate way of payment or payment for services which do not meet professional standards;

False and unnecessary prescription of medications;

Waiver of deduction and/or co-payment;

Running unnecessary medical services;

Provision of health care below standard level (e.g. m old people's homes); and

Failing to meet requests for the coverage of costs.

Patients may make false claims, and they can also inflate claims in cooperation with other actors in the health care system or on they own. Thus, they may offer money to health care providers to be issued with the necessary medical results, forge results from nonexistent medical institutions or pay multiple visits to different doctors in order to be given doctor's prescriptions for those medical devices and substances the distribution of which is systematically controlled (*doctor-shopping*). Users of medical services may also be part of criminal groups which engage in fraudulent acts in an organized manner, where they may stage an accident so as to be provided with appropriate health care or claim compensation from insurance companies. The payers of health services usually commit frauds during financial transactions. As it is the case with other types, the most common forms in these types of fraudulent acts are misrepresentation of information, conducting dishonest transactions, absence of contracts based on which the transactions are made etc.[300]

As it was mentioned above, employers in health-service and other institutions in the health care system may also be the perpetrators of fraudulent acts. The following occur as the most common forms of criminal acts: inadequate presentation of the number of employees, avoidance of paying for insurance policies, dissuading the employees from seeking medical assistance in case of illness and injury at work or outside the workplace, but also willful referring of employees to treatments with a view to obtaining benefits and other fees etc. Health-service organizations may also fix the receipt of medical equipment as well as its use, while it has actually never been received etc.

There are diverse examples of frauds committed by health care providers, material or equipment retailers. The forms of frauds in these cases are publishing and making of inaccurate claims, claims about altered products, medications counterfeiting, distribution of products which are not fit for use due to their expiry . What should also be mentioned is the instance of fraud which involves hiring unlicensed professionals as well as incompetent and unqualified persons to provide health services.

Health care frauds which originate from health services providers, i.e. medical staff, are the prototypes of fraudulent acts in the health care system. The most common examples are false claims about the services which have not been provided, followed by double claims, failure to report double payments, alternations or modifications of diagnosis or medical services codes, reports of services which were not rendered, charged examinations which have never been done.

---

300 ikolovski, S. op. cit., p. 517-548.

Moreover, doctors and other medical staff may offer money to healthy persons in exchange for their visits for unnecessary examinations, unnecessary surgical procedures may be done, services which are more expensive than those that were actually provided may be charged etc. Sometimes health services providers may team up in committing fraudulent acts with other participants (e.g. institutions which provide diagnostic services or pharmaceutical and medical devices or equipment manufacturers).[301]

Likewise, many actors in the health system may be involved in dishonest activities. Individuals who are not medically trained may perform medical activities and/or pass themselves off health care workers (quackery), criminal groups or individuals may trade in information on patients or health care providers, report false information and receive funding for medical services which have never been provided.[302]

---

301 Li J, Huang KY, J. Jin & J. Shi, *A survey on srarisrical methods for health care fraud derection.* Health Care Manage Sci. 11 :275-287 .,2008, doi: I 0.1007/s 10729-007-9045-4.
302 ikolovski, S. op.cit., p. 517-548.

11. CRIMINAL LAW AND CRIMINAL ASPECTS OF THE PROTECTION OF HUMAN HEALTH

In the Republic Of Serbia great attention is given to human health care, which is supported by the fact that the right to health care of each citizen is guaranteed by the Constitution and that a large number of laws has been adopted in the field of health care. Thus health care legislation is considered to be a special area. Criminal-law protection in this field is characterized by subsidiarity, since the protection of human health is primarily provided within branches of law, and fragmentariness, because it is provided for most serious forms of attacks and harms to human health.

The protection of health also has a great significance at an international and regional level, which is supported by a great number of adopted international and regional conventions and acts (e.g. International Covenant on Economic, Social and Cultural Rights, European Convention for the Protection of Human Rights and Fundamental Freedoms, European Convention for the Protection of Human Rights and Dignity of the Human Being with regard to the Application of Biology and Medicine, European Convention for the Protection of Human Rights, European Convention of Human Rights and Biomedicine, The European Social Charter, etc.)[303] where the human health is seen as one of the most important goods that enjoys legal protection.

The significance of the right to life and the right to health as its integral part imposes a need of its uttermost criminal-law protection, which not only incriminates various forms of doing or failing to do, that cause harm or endanger life, but also determines obligations of providing help in averting possible threat to human life. This represents the ultimate scope of criminal-law protection of the right to life.[304]

---

303 For more details please see: Ayala, A., et al. *Ljudska prava u zdravsrvenoj zastiti:* prirucnik za prakticare, University of Belgrade School of, 2015
304 Dordevic, D. *Neukazivanje lekarske pomoci,* Kazneno pravo i medicina, Tematski zbornik radova medunarodnog znacaja, Palic, 29th-30th May, 2019, Institut za kriminoloska i socioloska istrazivanja, Srbija, 2019, p.245-258.

Health workers, and especially doctors, while performing their daily duties, are exposed to the influence of various interests, which may raise the question of their responsibility. It is often a case in medical practice that patients or their family members try to gain certain (mostly material) personal advantage from alleged medical errors and their consequences in civil-law litigation. There are world known instances in which injured patients where paid enormous sums of money, which is far from reality in our actual socioeconomic situation. On the other hand, there are more and more judicial proceedings which put the question of responsibility of doctors is raised on the account of negligence and malpractice in their work.

We increasingly witness unwanted phenomena of the media, especially the press, presenting such instances in unnecessarily sensational way, making subjective and often premature judgements of doctors and other medical workers at the stage when their malpractice is yet to be proved in the judicial proceeding. Moreover, it often happens that people of no professional touch with the medicine express their opinion publicly and very critically on whether the doctors did their job properly. Such public stigmatization of doctors may have serious consequences on their professional activity. Namely, even if the accused doctor is found not guilty by virtue of the final judgement, such epilogue is usually preceded by long (sometimes years long) and, for the accused, very exhausting process of defending, which unjustly casts a lifelong stain on that doctor's professional career. Bearing the aforementioned in mind, the saying that "every patient is a potential plaintiff" becomes a part of reality which our doctors more and more often face with in their practice.[305]

Nowadays, when the development of medical science is at an extraordinary level and scientific achievements have reached unfathomable proportions, it may be expected to witness the obliteration of negative social phenomenon of quackery. The question is raised as to why quite the opposite happens - that certain people turn to quackery more and more often. This question

---

305 Savic S. *Krivicna dela u vezi sa obavljanjem lekarske delamosti*. Naucni casopis urgentne medicine - halo 94, Vol. 16. o. 2, 56. Beograd, 2010., p. 54-65

is justifiable to raise considering that it may be frequently heard in the media about the cases of quack doctors and many people having been cured by them. Quackery has been rooted in our society from ancient times, but its expansion took place in the 1990s when quack doctors even mass advertised in the media.[306]

The following text will be discussing criminal-law protection of human health, with the special emphasis on criminal offenses that protect human health from different actions (doing and omitting to do), which are connected with medical treatment and providing other medical services and which may be done both by a doctor and other health care workers (the criminal offenses of Medical Malpractice pursuant to Article 251 of the Criminal Code and Failure to Provide Medical Assistance pursuant to Article 253 of the Criminal Code) and other persons who treat patients or provide other medical services, but are not adequately qualified, i.e. do not have a degree in medicine or dentistry, have not graduates from a medical high school, etc. (the criminal offense of Quackery and Unlicensed Practice of Pharmacy pursuant to Article 254 of the Criminal Code). Following the analysis of criminal-law protection of human health in general, with special a special reference to the criminal offenses of medical malpractice, failure to provide medical assistance, quackery and unlicensed practice of pharmacy, we will look into criminal aspect of quackery as a negative social phenomenon in the times of fast development of medical science and profession.

CRIMINAL-LAW PROTECTION OF HUMAN HEALTH IN THE REPUBLIC OF SERBIA

The authors of this work discuss criminal offenses against human health according to the Criminal Code of The Republic of Serbia. The subject of criminal-law protection is human health - both individual and health of people as common (general) good. Even though some criminal offenses against human health are not statistically significant, the authors believe that such criminal offenses are significant in terms of protection of human health as one of the most important goods protected by criminal law.

---

306 Randelovic, V. *Krivicno delo nadrilekarstvo u teoriji i sudskoj praksi,* Pravni zivot, o. 9/2019, p.233-248.

Health[307] is certainly a part of the most significant group protective objects. The right to health care is also the constitutional right of people. It is primarily protected within other branches of law, while criminal-law protection is in fact of fragmented character in this field and is necessary to be provided only in cases of drastic threat or harm to human health. Breaches as torts are foreseen for the violation of some these standards, while the criminal offenses are foreseen for the most serious breaches, which involve endangerment or the violation of the protected object.[308]

Criminal procedure law should, or rather must, recognize true perpetrators of the criminal act, i.e. criminal offense, and reinforce **both special and general prevention** (that is, significance of pronounced sanctions for the very perpetrator of the criminal offense, but also for the others to whom it would never occur to do something like that or something similar after they have seen the example of the punished perpetrator) with the very help of proper criminal sanctions.

The common opinion and fact that may serve as an axiom is that a doctor treats and can only help a person who needs medical help. There is unbreakable bond between a doctor and a patient. Everything relies on trust and confidence. Trust in the expertise and conscientiousness of a doctor, and confidence in being cured and healing. A doctor has to provide a medical service and apply adequate devices and appropriate treatment. In case that a doctor does not act in that manner, problems which enter the field of the criminal law arise.[309]

In criminal proceedings, providers of medical services may appear as suspects or as aggrieved parties. In both cases the norms of the Criminal Code and the Criminal Procedure Law apply.[310]

Material provisions of the Criminal Code are foreseen in chapter 23 "Criminal Offenses against Human Health". This group of criminal offenses includes:[311]

---

307 According to the definition by the World Health Organization, health means "the state of complete physical, mental and social well-being and not merely the absence disease or infirmity", World Health Organization, Constitution, Basic documents, Forty-fifth edition, Supplement, October 2006, Preamble, available at: https://www.who.int/governance/eb/who _constitution_ en.pdf,
308 Stojanovic, Z. *Komentar Krivicnog Zakonika Republike Srbije*, Sluzbeni glasnik, Beograd, 20 1 7., p.807.
309 *Krstenic, J. Odnos lekara i pacijenta*, 09.04.2021. available at:
https://www.otvorenavratapravosudja.rs/teme/krivicno-pravo/uvod-u-pitanja-prava-i-zdravlja accessed on: 14. 02. 2022.
310 Criminal Procedure Law, *"the Official Gazelle of the Republic of Serbia"*, No. 72/2011, 101/2011, 121/2012, 32/2013, 45/2013, 55/2014, 35/2019, 27/2021 - Decision made by the Constitution Court and 62/2021 - Decision made by the Constitution Court.
311 Criminal Code *"the Official Gazelle of the Republic of Serbia"*, o. 85/2005, 88/2005 - corr., 107/2005 - corr., 72/2009, 111/2009, 121/2012, 104/2013, 108/2014, 94/2016 i 35/2019

unlawful production and circulation of narcotics (Article 246)
unauthorized possession of narcotics (Article 246a)
facilitating the taking of narcotics (Article 247)
failure to act pursuant to health regulations during epidemic (Article 248)
transmitting contagious disease (Article 249)
transmitting HIV infection (Article 250)
medical malpractice (Article 251)
illegal conducting of medical experiments and testing of drugs (Article 252)
failure to provide medical assistance (Article 253)
quackery and unlicensed practice of pharmacy (Article 254)
malpractice in preparing and issuing medicaments (Article 255)
production and putting in circulation of harmful products (Article 256)
unconscientious inspection of foodstuffs (Article 257)
pollution of drinking water and foodstuffs (Article 258)
grave offenses against health (Article 259)

A large number of criminal offenses against human health are formal and inchoate criminal offenses since they do not have a consequence as an element of the substance of the criminal offense, and thus are considered to be completed by the very undertaking of the act of execution (e.g. criminal act of quackery and unlicensed practice of pharmacy, Article 254 of the Criminal Code, etc.). In this regard, with the majority of criminal acts against human health the consequences assume abstract threat to human health which, at the same time, represent legal incrimination motive. It means that the act of commission itself is considered dangerous and that it is not allowed to prove the act could not have happened. Literature offers various criteria for the classification of criminal offenses against health. One classification criterion is according to the circumstance whether the consequence - the threat is or is not the element of crime. Another classification criterion is according to the characteristics of the perpetrator, that is whether it is a person who must possess certain characteristics or the perpetrator may be any person.[312] The classification is also possible according to what the human health is protected from:[313]

312 Tahovic, J. *Krivicino pravo*, Posebni deo, Savremena administracija, Beograd, 1961, p. 246-24 7.
313 Randelovic, V. op.cit., p.233-248.

e) Grave offenses against health comprise a special group pursuant to Article 259 of the Criminal Code, which comprises qualified forms of the majority of criminal offenses against human health. these criminal offenses are prescribed by common provisions pursuant to Article 259 of the Criminal Code due to legislative technique, i.e. in order to avoid repetition. Premeditated forms of these criminal offenses are included in paragraphs I and 2, where there must be negligence in relation to a more severe consequence, which includes grave bodily harm, a serious health impairment or death of one or more persons.

Unintentional forms of these criminal offenses are contained in paragraphs 3 and 4, and in relation to a more severe consequence, which also means grave bodily harm, serious health impairment or death of one or more persons, where there must be negligence.

Criminal offenses which belong to the group of offenses against health, beside common protected object, have no other common characteristics. This indicates that protection of human health is a very wide area. It could be said they have similarities with criminal offenses against general safety of people and property as they, as a rule, cause danger to an unspecified number of people or large number of people. According to consequences which ensued, these criminal offenses have some similarities with offenses against life and body. However, the differ from each other by specific circumstances and modi operandi.

Criminal offenses from the group of criminal offenses against health are *delicta propria,* which means that a particular characteristic of the perpetrator presents important characteristic of the substance of the criminal offense (criminal offense of medical malpractice pursuant to Article 251 of the Criminal Code, criminal offense of failure to provide medical assistance pursuant to Article 253 of the Criminal Code, criminal offense of malpractice in preparing and issuing medicaments pursuant to Article 255 of the Criminal Code and criminal offense of unconscientious inspection of the foodstuffs pursuant to Article 257 of the Criminal Code) and therefore these criminal offenses are considered as separate crimes. That means that the perpetrator may only be a particular person with a particular characteristic, e.g., a doctor, pharmacist, veterinarian, while a perpetrator of other criminal offenses from this group may be any person, and therefore they belong to the group of general criminal offenses, which means that the perpetrator may be every person which the law recognizes as an active subject of the criminal offense, i.e., a perpetrator may be any person (e.g. quackery or unlicensed practice of pharmacy pursuant to Article 254 of the Criminal Code, unlawful production and circulation of Narcotics pursuant to Article 246 of the Criminal Code, etc.)

Majority of criminal offenses from Chapter 23 of the Criminal Code have a blanket disposition. It means that the Criminal Code does not determine the content of the criminal offense on the whole in its description, but refers to other regulations supplementary to the disposition. That is, a large number of criminal offenses against human health has a blanket character since it is stated in the legal description that the punishable behavior means a breach of certain regulations, which are usually part of health legislation (e.g., criminal offense of failure to provide medical assistance pursuant to Article 253 of the Criminal Code etc.). Criminal Code defines all characteristics of a particular criminal offense. However, the content of one of the legal signs is defined by another regulation. Great number of criminal offenses in this chapter represent premeditated criminal offenses. Some of them are punishable if committed as a result of negligence[314] (e.g., medical malpractice pursuant to Article 251 of the Criminal Code).

On this occasion, some criminal offenses will be analyzed in more detail within criminal-law protection of human health, which legally sanctions irregular work of doctors and other medical workers in the process of medical treatment: medical malpractice (pursuant to Article 251), failure to provide medical assistance (pursuant to Article 253), criminal offense of quackery and unlicensed practice of pharmacy (pursuant to Article 254) will be analyzed, the perpetrator of which may be any person recognized by law as an active subject of the criminal offense, i.e., any person, without adequate professional qualifications, who provides treatment or other medical services or prepares or issues medicaments, while misusing the trust of people whose health is impaired or endangered and who expect adequate medical assistance - intervention, request a medicament and expect that medicament to help them.

---

314 When we say that someone commits an offense as a result of negligence, that means that that person is aware that he or she may commit an office, but he or she reckle sly a sumes that it would not happen or that he or she will be able to prevent, or when that person is not aware that he or she may commit an offense by his or her action although he or she was obliged to be and could be aware of that possibility according to the circumstances under which such offense was committed and according to his or her personal characteristics.(*Krstenic, J. Odnos lekara i pacijenta,* 09.04.2021. available at: https://www.otvorenavratapravosudja.rs/teme/k.rivicno-pravo/uvod-u-pitanja-prava-i-zdravlja, accessed on: 14. 02. 2022)

Medical Malpractice

> ### Medical Malpractice
> ### Article 251
>
> A doctor who in providing medical services uses an evidently inadequate means or an evidently unsuitable treatment or fails to observe appropriate hygiene standards or evidently acts unconscientiously and thereby causes deterioration of a person's health, shall be punished by imprisonment of three months to three years.
>
> The penalty specified in paragraph 1 of this Article shall be imposed to other medical staff who in rendering medical assistance or care or performing other medical activity proceeds in an obviously unconscientious manner thereby causing deterioration of a person's medical condition.
>
> If the offense specified in paragraphs 1 and 2 of this Article are committed from negligence, the offender shall be punished by fine or imprisonment up to one year.

Human health is foreseen as an important object of protection by criminal legislation. Although the aim in the work of each doctor as well as other health care workers is the improvement of health and patient's healing, sometimes the cases of medical errors occur.[315] Like all the other professionals, doctors may and do make mistakes in their work, but it should be emphasized that not each mistake in the work of a doctor can be declared medical malpractice in criminal-legal sense. Without going into theoretical debate on the definition of the term of medical error in legal and medical sense, the definition of professional error according to the LHC will be quoted. [316] Professional error means "unconscientious performance of health

---

315 When transposed to the filed of criminal law, the colloquial term medical error, which is often used in the media, refers, above all, to the criminal offense of medical malpractice pursuant to Article 251 of the Criminal Code, but it also refers to more serious forms of this criminal offense which is foreseen by Article 259 of the Criminal Code and named grave offenses against human health. (Pavlovic., B., Markovic, I., Cetkovic, P. *Pravo na zdravstvenu zastitu kroz prizmu lekarske greske,* Ju titia, Ca opis udruzenja sudijskih i tuzilackih pomocnika Srbije, br. l /20 l 6, p. 18-21.)

316 Article 186, the Law on Health Care, *"the Official Gazelle of the Republic of Serbia"* No. 25/2019.

care, carelessness or omission, i.e. failing to conform to the established rules of profession and professional skills in providing health care, which leads to injury, damage, deterioration of health or loss of parts of a patient's body". The criminal offense of medical malpractice is defined in Article 251 of the Criminal Code (Chapter 23 - Criminal offenses against Human Health).[317]

In health care, efficient, correct, professional and timely provision of a health service, e.g. medical assistance, as well as the performance of any other health care activity, e.g. provision of medical care, are of particular significance. Thereby, the social function is realized as well as the protection of the rights to inviolability of physical and mental integrity and to human health, which are guaranteed by the Constitution. In that regard it should be underlined that there is a possibility that a certain doctor's activity or other medical activity may result in the deterioration of health of the person who was the subject of that activity. In case this is the matter of gross/grave violation of doctor's or other medical duty, i.e the case of gross violation of the rules of medical profession, as a result of which serious consequences for the health of another person or other persons ensue, all types of legislation foresee criminal liability and punishment for a particular criminal offense - medical malpractice.

Correct treatment of people, i.e. the treatment which is in line with the rules of medical science and medical profession is of utmost importance in each society. This is ensured by various means, ranging from from the doctor's code and ethical standards, administrative law in health care, to damages in civil law in case of medical malpractice. One of the means is also criminal law, which has very limited possibilities in this area and it should really be ultima ratio.[318]

The criminal offense has two main forms which differ according to who a perpetrator can be.[319]

---

317 Savic, S. Znacaj *sudskomedicinskog vestacenja u slucajevima krivicnog dela nesavesnog pruianja lekarske pomoci*, Kazneno pravo i medicina, Tematski zbomik radova medunarodnog znacaja, Pa lie, 29th-30th May 2019., Institute for Criminal and Sociological Research, Serbia, 2019, p.259-274.
318 *Ultimo ratio* character of the criminal law arise from the principle of legitimacy and it is partially defined by Article of the Criminal Code of the Republic of Serbia, which stipulates that "Protection of a human being and other fundamental social values constitute the basis and scope for defining of criminal acts, imposing of criminal sanctions and their enforcement to a degree necessary for suppression of these of Tenses." Banovic, J. *Ultimo ratio karakter krivicnog prava u svetlu krivicnog dela Gradenje bez gradevinske dozvole* (cl. 219a KZ). Crimen (Beograd), I 0(1), 2019., p. 69-86. available at: https://doi.org/ 10.5937/crimen1901069B
319 Stojanovic, Z. op. cit., p.809.

The perpetrators of this criminal offense may be doctors (of medicine or of dental medicine) (paragraph 1) as well as all other health care workers (paragraph 2) and this is what the first and second basic form of this criminal offense differ in. The status of the doctor is not of significance as it can be a doctor working on the basis of an employment contract, a doctor who is an intern, but also a retired doctor. What is important for the commission of this criminal offense is that the doctor in the concrete case is performing a duty which involves the provision medical assistance.[320]

The act of commission of the first basic form is postulated alternatively and it exists when a doctor, in providing medical assistance, does the following: 1) applies a means which is evidently inadequate; 2) gives the treatment which is evidently unsuitable; 3) does not apply the appropriate hygienic measures; 4) or generally acts unconscientiously. It is important to underline that these actions must be undertaken in the course of providing medical assistance, i.e. treatment, which includes establishing the diagnosis and determining and implementing therapy.

The term "means of medical treatment" comprises all "the means which are taken into body or placed on the body for the purpose of establishing a diagnosis or treatment or for preventative reasons". The "method of treatment" represents the method which is applied in diagnostics and treatment.[321] The application of an evidently inadequate means or evidently unsuitable method of treatment involves all activities in the work of a doctor where there is evident and drastic departure from valid and generally accepted principles of medical science and practice, i.e. anything which represents a conspicuous mistake which is outside the framework of medical tolerance. Taking into consideration all the aforementioned facts, what can be considered to be an evidently inadequate means of treatment in practice is, for instance, penicillin administered to a person in whose medical records it is decidedly stated that he or she is allergic to this antibiotic, or giving transfusion of blood of the wrong type. An evidently unsuitable method of treatment is, for example, the decision that a patient diagnosed with the ruptured spleen with abdominal haemorrhage should be treated conservatively, and not surgically, i.e. by being subjected to splenectomy.[322]

---

320 Savic, S. op.cit., p.259-274.
321 Ibidem.
322 Savic S. op.cit., p. 54-65.

An evidently inadequate means of treatment involves the means which, according to the rules of medical profession, is not intended for the treatment of a certain illness and which can have a detrimental effect instead of curing. If it is administered to a patient for curing a certain illness, while that patient has another illness which is deteriorated by the administration of that means, inadequacy exists if the effects of contraindication prevail over the effect of indication. A very high level of inadequacy must be present here. It is for that reason that the word "evidently" is used as it is the matter of a conspicuous doctor's mistake by which he or she grossly violates the rules of medical science and profession.[323]

Another form of the act of commission is an evidently inappropriate method of treatment. This act is fairly similar to the application of an evidently inadequate means and in some cases a means and a method cannot be considered separately, i.e. isolated from one another. However, a method of treatment is a wider term and it denotes both the manner in which a means for treatment is used and some other procedures and treatments with the aim of curing patients, which may be done even without administering a certain means to a patient. In medical literature, the term "a method of treatment" means the method which is applied in diagnostics and in treatments. A very high level of unsuitability of the method of treatment has to be present here as well.

The next and the third form of the act of commission of this criminal offense is failure to implement appropriate hygienic measures. Medical profession sets certain standards in terms of hygienic measures, which may be of general and specific character (e.g. surgical procedures require complete sterility). This form of the act of commission may also occur as an act of commission of the form of this criminal offense foreseen by paragraph 2 as complying with and implementing hygienic measures is a duty present with other health care workers as well. Therefore, in addition to doctors, co-perpetrators in the concrete case may also be other health care workers. Failure to implement the appropriate hygienic measures as a form negligence may also relate to, for example, inadequate preparation of a surgeon/nurse-medical technician or an operating area, which is not in accordance with the standards/principle of asepsis and antisepsis in surgery.

---

323 Savic, D. *Krivicna dela protiv zdravlja ljudi,* December 20th, 2017, available at: https://nomcentarngo.com/krivicna-dela-protiv-zdravlja-ljudi/ accessed on: 14. 02. 2022.

What follows is the fourth form of the act of commission which is defined relatively through the formulation "or evidently acts unconscientiously." This typically means failure to apply an evidently adequate means or it may be the case of general negligence which is not characteristic of the procedure of treatment only. In health care practice, one of the possible form of unconscientious acting is also inadequate keeping of medical documents, which unfortunately happens more and more often in our practice. It happens that the medical history of a patient who passed away after having been treated for several days or even several weeks contain only the findings recorded at the admittance and the conclusion on the fatal outcome, without any data on the course of the illness, i.e. the state of the patient during the course of treatment. One of the relatively frequent examples is also failure to keep the anesthetic records up to date with surgical interventions conducted under general anesthesia, which creates great problems in the subsequent forensic medical expertise in case the patient dies while being under general anesthesia.[324]

While in the first case it can be acknowledged that there is an act of commission of this criminal offense (when a doctor omits to use an evidently appropriate means or treatment procedure), the second case arouses certain dilemmas. Nevertheless, the higher level of negligence is required here as well. Bearing in mind that the first two forms of the act of commission are the matter of gross violation of medical profession, and that some room is left for a medical error, the existence of the higher level of negligence is necessary here as well. This is more so as the term "evidently unconscientious in general" may include rather heterogeneous situations and even atypical cases where the possibility of error is more likely. The law explicitly requires the higher level of negligence here as well, which corresponds to the notion of incrimination, and in that respect it is also harmonized with other forms of the acts of commission which require higher level of negligence.[325]

The consequence of this criminal offense pursuant to paragraph 1 involves the deterioration of the health condition of a person, which has to be caused by one of the mentioned forms of the acts of commission.

---

324 Savic S. op.cit., p. 54-65
325 Stojanovic, Z. op.cit., p.810.

The second form of this criminal offense pursuant to paragraph 2 differs from the form defined in paragraph 1 only by a perpetrator, and that can be any health care worker, i.e. a person who performs certain tasks within the provision of medical assistance or in the area of another health care activity, but who is not a doctor. For the act of commission to be present, that person has to act with evident negligence, which must result in the deterioration of the health condition of a person. In this case, the act of commission is adjusted to it, i.e. this is not the matter of treatment, but of providing medical assistance or care or performing another health care activity, while for the presence of the act of commission, it is necessary that the perpetrator has acted with evident negligence in performing those activities. Here, as it is the case with paragraph 1, the presence of milder forms of negligence is not sufficient. With this form as well as with the form defined in paragraph 1, the rules in health care may be of significance in establishing the notion of negligence, apart from disregard for certain rules of medical science and profession. There is an important provision contained in Article 48 of the LHC, which stipulates that, in providing health care, a health-service institution and private practice are obliged to apply scientifically proven, verified and safe health care technologies in the prevention, diagnostics, treatments, medical care and rehabilitation of the ill and the injured[326] as well as to apply only those methods and complementary medicine procedures which are allowed.[327]

With this form as well with the form of the offense pursuant to paragraph 1, the consequence of the criminal offense is the deterioration of the health condition of a person caused by the act of commission.

As for culpability for the forms pursuant to paragraphs 1 and 2, premeditation is required. Considering the nature of the criminal offense, it has to be possible premeditation. It should include personal unconscientious action as well as the consent to the consequence. If there were direct premeditation, another criminal offense would be in question depending on the gravity and the kind of the consequences caused.

---

326 Article 48 of Law on Health Care, "the Official Gazelle of the Republic of Serbia" o.25/2019
327 Ibid., Article 218.

Grave offenses against human health pursuant to Article 259 of the Criminal Code are qualified forms of the criminal offense pursuant to Article 251 of the Criminal Code as well as of other criminal offenses from the set of the criminal offenses against human health. Criminal offenses qualified by a graver consequence as defined by Article 27 of the Criminal Code are in question. All the criminal offenses concern the same consequences, which are regulated by the provisions of the same article for legislative technique. Article 259 foresees more severe punishment in cases in which medical malpractice caused the ensuing of graver consequences in the form of grave bodily harm, serious health impairment or the death of a patient.

As regards the criminal offense of medical malpractice, paragraph 3 foresee a involuntary form which is different from the first forms in terms of culpability and for which a milder punishment is foreseen. Advertent and inadvertent negligence are possible. With the former, a perpetrator is aware that he or she acts negligently, i.e. that he or she fails to act in accordance with the rules of medical profession, but he or she recklessly assumes that the consequence will not ensue, while with inadvertent negligence, there is no such awareness, but there is a possibility and duty to foresee the ensuing of the consequence. Thus, there is the involuntary form of this criminal offense (qualified by a graver consequence) which has been committed due to advertent negligence in the case when an anesthesiologist did not provide the sufficient quantity of oxygen during the operation at the moment when a patient was being subjected to general anesthesia by having the breathing tube improperly positioned as a consequence of which breathing difficulties ensued, resulting in the death of the patient (OSB Kz. 3053/03).[328]

It is very important to establish the existence of the causal relationship between medical malpractice and the ensuing harmful consequence.[329] In this regard, it should be proven conclusively that the deterioration of the health condition has been caused by the very negligence of a doctor, i.e. that it has not been the result of the very nature of the primary disease, injury or other factors which were mentioned previously when the term of an accident was explained (specific circumstances of a case, personal characteristic and particular conditions of the patient's body).[330]

---

328 Stojanovic, Z. op. cit., p. 812.
329 Savic, D. *Krivicna dela proriv zdravlja ljudi* available at http ://nomcentamgo.com/krivicna-dela-protiv-zdravlja-ljudi/ visited on: 14.02.2022.
330 Savic S. op. cit., p. 54-65.

The essence of this criminal offense comes down to the fact that in each concrete case it should be examined whether the doctor or another medical worked acted *lege artis* or *contra lege*. The consent of an ill person does exclude the culpability of a doctor or another medical worker in providing medical assistance. The consequences may be reflected in grave bodily injury or grave impairment of health of a passive subject or even the death of one or more persons. Proper medical treatment of people, i.e. medical treatment which is in accordance with the rules of medical profession and science is of utmost importance in every society. This concerns a criminal offense in the instance of which criminal law and medicine overlap, i.e. the expectations from two sides - patients and their doctors - meet. On one side there are patients who are usually uninformed of their health condition and thus they put great trust in doctors and other medical staff, whereas on the other side there are doctors who often feel unjustifiably stigmatized as the very nature of their profession bears the risk from medical error, which is often publicly presented with unnecessary sensationalism. Medical profession is in the very top by the level of professional liability and the gravest violation of the requirements of the profession which are so highly set are foreseen as criminal offenses.[331]

The aforementioned leads to the conclusion that the criminal offense of medical malpractice pursuant to Article 251 of the Criminal Code is, above all, committed by a doctor who, in providing medical assistance, applies an evidently inadequate means or an evidently unsuitable method of treatment or fails to apply the appropriate hygienic measures or generally acts with evident negligence and thus causes the deterioration of the health condition of a person.

Negligent work of doctors does not necessarily cause the deterioration of the patient's state in all cases. If a doctor acts negligently, but such an act does not result in a harmful consequence in the form of the deterioration of the health condition of a person, there will be no elements for the criminal prosecution of that doctor (e.g. when the doctor does not prescribe an appropriate antibiotic in the case of proven streptococcal pharyngitis, but the infection heals spontaneously regardless of that and without harmful effects on the patient). However, the absence of elements of criminal liability in such

---

331 Pavlovic., B., Markovic, I., Cetkovic, P. op.cit., p.18-21.

cases certainly does not mean that a doctor should not assume certain professional responsibility for the proven negligence in accordance with the nature of the criminal offense committed, which is nowadays reflected in losing a licence (permit) for practicing medicine worldwide.[332]

In Serbia professional sanctioning by the Serbian Medical Chamber is foreseen for doctors' negligence in parallel to criminal-law punishment. Professional liability of a doctor for a professional error is established in disciplinary proceedings before the competent authority of the Serbian Medical Chamber, within regular and exceptional professional work quality checks proceedings as well as in other proceedings defined by law.[333]

The LHC no longer foresees the possibility of permanent, but only of temporary revocation of licence if a doctor has been convicted of premeditated criminal offense by virtue of a final court decision and sentenced to six months' imprisonment or was given a more severe sentence or if he or she was sentenced to imprisonment for the criminal offense against human health, and the temporary revocation of licence may last until the deletion of the conviction in accordance with the Criminal Code. Thus, one of the legal reasons for the revocation of medical licence is the final decision on the imprisonment sentence for any criminal offense against human health contained in Chapter 23 of the Criminal Code, including the criminal offense pursuant to Article 251 of the Criminal Code. The aforementioned leads to the conclusion that the temporary revocation of licence is foreseen for a doctor who has been sentenced to six months' imprisonment or was given a more severe sentence for any premeditated criminal offense, while the form of guilt, i.e. whether a criminal offense has been premeditated or involuntary is not stated for criminal offenses against human health.[334]

---

332 Savic S. op.cit., p. 54-65.
333 The Law on Health Care, "the Official Gazette of the Republic of Serbia" No.25/2019
334 Savic, S. op. cit., p.259-274.

Failure to Provide Medical Assistance

Failure to Provide Medical Assistance
Article 253

A doctor who contrary to his duty refuses to render medical assistance to a person in need of such assistance, and whose life is in immediate and present danger or is in danger of onset of grave bodily harm or serious deterioration of health, shall be punished by fine or imprisonment up to two years.

If due to the offense specified in paragraph 1 of this Article, the person to whom medical assistance was not provided sustains grave bodily harm or serious deterioration of health, the offender shall be punished by imprisonment of six months to five years.

If the offense specified in paragraph 1 of this Article results in death of the person to whom medical assistance was not provided, the offender shall be punished by imprisonment of one to eight years.

A doctor is obliged to examine a person in all situations and to ascertain that person's present state of health by the examination, so if the doctor establishes the presence of immediate danger to that person's life or from the onset of grave bodily harm or grave impairment of health, he or she is obliged to render medical assistance in accordance with the possibilities presently at his or her disposal in that concrete situation. In practice, a doctor may find him- or herself in situations in which he or she has to take care of several injured or ill persons at the same time and then the level of a threat to life is the main criterion based on which a doctor should establish the order in which he or she would provide assistance. In other words, a doctor may leave a patient he or she taking care of if that patient's life is not threatened at that moment and his or her illness or injury may be adequately treated by the doctor subsequently.[335]

---

335 Ayala, A., i dr. op. cit.,str.326.

Breach of medical duty to provide medical assistance may have grave consequences on the health and life of people. For that reason and in certain circumstances, it may present grounds not only for professional and moral responsibility, but also for criminal liability. One of the criminal offenses by which this kind of a doctor's responsibility is established in our Criminal Code is also the criminal offense of failure to provide medical assistance. Although it is relatively rare in judicial practice, this criminal offense is important from the aspect of the protection of human life and health and for the establishment of a doctor's responsibility.

The criminal offense of failure to provide medical assistance pursuant to Article 253 of the Criminal Code has a basic form (paragraph 1) and two qualified forms (paragraphs 2 and 3).

The act of commission of the basic form (paragraph 1) involves the doctor's refusal to provide medical assistance to a person in need of such assistance, and whose life is in imminent danger or in danger of the onset of grave bodily harm or serious impairment of health.

Although this is not explicitly specified by the law, the danger from the onset of grave bodily harm or serious impairment of health must be immediate (as it is the case with a threat to life). Refusal in case of this criminal offense does not have to be explicit. Premeditated omission to provide medical assistance is sufficient. Starting from the aim of this incrimination, it can be said that medical assistance involves only the assistance which is necessary for the removal of immediate threat to life or from the onset of a grave bodily harm or serious impairment of health. This concerns the act of failure to take action (omission). The duty to act derives from the very medical profession as well as from the relevant regulations (e.g. from the Law on Health Care). The legal description of this criminal offense concretizes that duty as it requires that the refusal should be done "contrary to the duty in the given moment", and not contrary to a doctor's duty in general. That means that all circumstances must be taken into consideration in the given case so that it could be assessed whether a doctor in the concrete situation failed to act contrary to his or her duty. The question in that regard is whether that duty means that medical assistance should be provided at any time and in any place. In principle, the answer to this question should be affirmative, but in each concrete case it is necessary to establish whether a doctor was able to provide such assistance.[336]

The failure to provide medical assistance does not necessarily have to result in the death or impairment of the health of a person whose life was in immediate danger for the basic form of this criminal offense (quoted in paragraph 1 of Article 253 of the Criminal Code) to be present. In other words, a perpetrator will be punished by law even if the person to whom medical assistance was not provided survives without any detrimental consequences on the health. Paragraphs 2 and 3 of Article 253 of the Criminal Code, however, foresee a more severe punishment for a doctor if the failure to provide medical assistance results in harmful consequences in the form of grave bodily harm, serious impairment of health or in the death of a person who was not provided with medical assistance[337] (e.g. A doctor failed to provide assistance to an injured person on the pretext that the institution he or she works for was not on call at that moment or in charge of receiving patients.). Thus, in comparison to medical malpractice, in this case the detrimental consequence does not necessarily ensues.

In the text that follows, we will show an interesting comparison of the criminal offense of failure to provide medical assistance pursuant to Article 253 of the Criminal Code to the criminal offense of failure to render aid pursuant to Article 127 of the Criminal Code.

Failure to Render Aid

Article 127

Whoever fails to render aid to a person in life-threatening situation although he could have done so without risk to himself or another, shall be punished with fine or imprisonment up to two years.

If failure to render aid results in serious health impairment or other grievous bodily harm of the person in life-threatening situation, the offender shall be punished with fine or imprisonment up to three years.

---

336 Stojanovic, Z. op. cit., p. 814-815
337 Savic S. op. cit., p. 54-65

255

(3) If failure to render aid results in death of the person in life-threatening situation, the offender shall be punished with imprisonment of three months to five years.

Article 127 mentions the criminal liability of other persons, who are not doctors, for failure to render assistance to a person in immediate life-threatening situation. For these persons ("who are not doctors) the law foresees the obligation of rendering assistance only if it could be done without putting oneself or another person in danger. Conversely, in Article 253, which refers to doctors, there is no such restriction, which leads to the conclusion that a doctor is legally obliged to provide assistance to a person in an immediate life-threatening danger even if he or she would put him- or herself in danger. In practice, the criminal-law consideration of such situations mainly refers to cases when a doctor refuses to provide assistance to a person suffering from a serious contagious disease (AIDS, hepatitis B and C) for fear of getting infected during such intervention.[338]

The passive subject of the criminal offense of failure to provide medical assistance pursuant to Article 253, i.e. the object of action is the person who is in need of medical assistance and who is in immediate life-threatening danger or in danger of the onset of grave bodily harm or grave impairment of health. That means that both of these two conditions must be cumulatively satisfied, i.e. that apart from the presence of immediate danger, a person who is in such danger is in need of medical assistance for the removal of that danger. Namely, it is possible that someone may be in immediate life-threatening danger or in danger of the onset of grave bodily harm or serious health impairment for some other reasons and not for a disease or injury, in which case that person does not need medical assistance. Although the legal description in that regard is not completely clear, danger from the onset of grave bodily harm or serious impairment of health must be immediate as well.[339]

The perpetrator (subject) of this criminal offense is exclusively the very doctor who refuses to provide medical assistance, either by refusing to do so directly or by hiding his or her identity, i.e.

---

338 Ayala, A., et al. op. cit., p.327.
339 Stojanovic, Z. op. cit.,p. 815.

the work he or she does (e.g. A doctor in the street notices that a person has been injured in a traffic accident, but he or she leaves the scene of the accident nonetheless, without attempting to provide assistance to the injured person). Failure to provide medical assistance represents the typical example of so called *delicta propria,* i.e. criminal offenses with which a perpetrator has to have a certain quality. Article 253 of the Criminal Code, which defines this criminal offense, mentions a doctor as a perpetrator of this offense. Although the term of *doctor* seems generally known at first glance, the impression is that it is this very element which could be appear before all as disputable with this criminal offense.340

This term is neither defined in the very prov1s10n on this criminal offense (or the provision on the criminal offense of medical malpractice, where a doctor also figures as a perpetrator) in the Criminal Code nor is it defined in Article 112, in which the meaning of certain terms used in the Criminal Code are defined.

The Criminal Code does not specify which doctor this criminal offense relates to, which in theory means that it sanctions any doctor regardless of the kind of activity he or she performs, i.e. his or her present capability to provide adequate medical assistance.

In that regard, it is disputable whether a perpetrator can be any doctor or only the one who practices medicine, i.e. who is engaged in that profession. In principle, any doctor can be a potential perpetrator, but with doctors who do not practice medicine (i.e. who have the required professional qualifications, but perform other similar or completely different work or are retired etc.) it should be specifically examined whether the condition that they have acted "contrary to their medical duty" is met. For example, a professor at the university of medicine (depending on the subject he lectures on or whether he practices medicine) could still be considered a perpetrator of this criminal offense if he or she would fail to provide medical assistance. However, the one who has never practiced medicine and has another job (e.g. a sales specialist in a company selling medical devices and equipment) never has such a duty and thus he or she could not be a perpetrator of this criminal offense even though that person is a doctor by profession. That, however, means that the narrower interpretation of the term *doctor* is only justified here. The aim of incrimination is to incriminate

---

340 Dordevic, D. op.cit., p.245-258.

the refusal of medical assistance by a person who is capable of providing such assistance, for which it would not be sufficient that that person has a university degree in medicine, but that he or she also practices (or practiced) medicine.[341]

This criminal offense does not comprise those cases where a doctor has examined a patient in the best possible way, but failed to established the presence of the life-threatening condition for certain circumstances (e.g. atypical clinical picture, unavailability of necessary diagnostic means). These situations could be classified under previously explained medical errors (in the medical sense of that term) by their character. The Criminal Code does not specify which doctor this criminal offense refers to, which in theory means that it sanctions any doctor, regardless of the work he or she performs, i.e. his or her capability to provide adequate medical assistance. This is practically the question as to whether a doctor who has worked in a research laboratory and outside medical practice for years would be capable of providing such assistance. Thus, the opinion that this criminal offense should relate only to doctors who practice medicine in health care organizations prevails in legal literature because the assistance should be real in relation to the concrete case.[342]

Paragraph 2 defines a more serious form of this criminal offense. It is required that an offense defined in paragraph 1 resulted in grave injury or serious impairment of health of the person who was not provided with medical assistance. This concerns a criminal offense qualified by a graver consequence and thus the provisions of Article 27 apply in relation to it. The most serious form is foreseen (paragraph 3), which exists in the case when the person who has not been provided with medical assistance dies. The provision of Article 27 is also applied here, i.e. it is required that the perpetrator acted with negligence in regard to the graver consequence.[343]

The major problems related to this criminal offense, above all, concern a potential perpetrator of this criminal offense, i.e. the term of *doctor* and the type and scope of assistance a doctor is obliged to provide as well as the level of endangerment of a passive subject who imposes the the obligation of the provision of assistance on the perpetrator.

---

341 Stojanovic, Z. op. cit., p.816.
342 Savic S. op. cit., p. 54-65.
343 Stojanovic, Z. op. cit., p. 8 I 6.

> **Quackery and Unlicensed Practice of Pharmacy**
>
> Quackery and Unlicensed Practice of Pharmacy
> **Article 254**
>
> Whoever without appropriate qualifications engages in providing medical treatment or rendering other medical services, shall be punished by fine or up to three years' imprisonment.
>
> (2) The penalty specified in paragraph 1 of this Article shall be imposed on whoever without proper qualifications engages in preparing or issuing of medicaments.

In the contemporary age, which is characterized by a high level of development of medical sciences, quackery is mostly assessed as a socially harmful phenomenon by the society, while the activities of the state authorities are directed towards suppressing this phenomenon. One of the consequences of these circumstances is defining quackery as a criminal offense in the legislation of a large number of modern countries. Human health represents a very important group object of protection in the criminal legislation of the Republic of Serbia.

The Criminal Code also defines the criminal offense of quackery and unlicensed practice of pharmacy in Article 254, within the group of criminal offenses against human health. Bearing in mind subsidiarity and fragmentariness as the basic features of the criminal law, according to which the criminal-law protection is given only when other branches of law cannot provide sufficiently effective protection and only to the most valuable goods as protection against the most serious attacks, the stance of the legislator that quackery represent a phenomenon which is a threat to human health and that the criminal-law protection of people is necessary in that sense is also clear.[344] As quackery represents a criminal offense against human health, it is perfectly clear that the legislator considers this criminal offense to be one of the most dangerous forms of attacks on human health.

---

344 Randelovic, V. op.cit., p.233-248.

Although quackery and unlicensed practice of pharmacy were foreseen as two criminal offenses in our previous legislation, this two incriminating acts are connected and defined in one article of the valid Criminal Code for the similarity and legislative technique. Namely, due to legislative technique as well as for the similarity between the criminal offense of quackery and unlicensed practice of pharmacy, these two criminal offenses are foreseen by the same Article 254.

The act of commission of the criminal offenses of quackery (paragraph 1) is defined alternatively and it includes either engaging in medical treatment or engaging in the provision of other medical services by a person without proper qualifications for such engagement. Although there are opinions to the contrary, in our theory there is still a view that a collective criminal offense is in question and earlier judicial practice accepted that view. That means that all individual criminal offenses are considered to be one criminal offense (apparent real concurrence), the consequence of which, among other things, is that "a conviction may not comprise those criminal offenses from its composition which have become statute-barred" (*VSS Kz. I 478/86*). With this criminal offense, however, it is important to establish the notion of engaging, while the construction of collective criminal offenses appears here as well as in general as excessive and obsolete.[345] For the notion of engaging it is not enough that the an act has been committed only once. If it has been committed only once, then there is no act of commission of this criminal offense (and there is no need for the construction of a collective criminal offense, i.e. the question of real or apparent real concurrence[346] is not raised). The view present in one part of our theory that it is sufficient for a collective criminal offense to exist that an offense has been committed only once if there is readiness to repeat that criminal offense is also unacceptable for the reason that one cannot be punished for his potential or future acts.[347]

---

345 Stojanovic, Z. op.cit., p. 817.
346 The concurrence of criminal offenses exists when one person commits several criminal offenses and he is tried for all those offenses at the same time. One verdict is passed and one sentence is pronounced. Several criminal offenses may be committed concurrently by the same perpetrator with one act-ideal concurrence of criminal offenses, but a criminal offense can also be committed by the same perpetrator with several acts committed at different times - real concurrence of criminal offenses. Concurrence may comprise two or more criminal offenses, while if the same criminal offenses are in question, there i homogeneous concurrence, and if different criminal offenses are in question, there is heterogeneous concurrence. Both of them can be both ideal and real concurrence. There is apparent ideal concurrence of criminal offense when is appears that several criminal offenses have been committed with one act, while there is in fact only one critninal offense. There is apparent real concurrence of cri1ninal offen es when it appears that several criminal offenses have been committed with several acts, while only one has actually been committed.
347 Stojanovic, Z. op.cit., p. 817.

Medical treatment involves all those activities which are generally undertaken by a doctor and they include establishing the diagnosis and deciding on therapy. It is thought that in certain circumstances the very establishing if the diagnosis, without determining therapy, cannot be considered medical treatment in the sense of this criminal offense, while administering medications or other substances or giving advice on medical treatment, without making the diagnosis, is always considered to be medical treatment in the sense of this incrimination. Providing medical services involves all those activities which may not be subsumed under medical treatment and which are undertaken by some other persons, such as, for instance, nurses, midwives, caregivers etc. Although it is sometimes hard to set the boundary, i.e. to establish whether an act represents medical treatment or provision of other medical services, it should be assumed that medical treatment includes all those activities generally done by a doctor, and provision of other medical services includes activities done by other health care workers.[348]

Medical treatment and provision of medical assistance represent an act of commission of this criminal offense even when this act is done in accordance with the requirements and rules of medical science. It is crucial that that an act of treatment or provision of medical assistance is done by a person without the required qualifications. A problem in particular regarding the act of commission are the acts and actions which belong to so-called alternative medicine as the persons who practice it, as a rule, do not have proper qualifications for giving medical treatment or providing medical assistance. If it were assumed that some of these actions represented medical treatment (e.g. bioenergy healing), there would be an act of commission of this criminal offense, regardless of the fact that incriminating such actions is politically dubious if such actions are harmless.[349]

The consequence of the criminal offense of quackery as well as of the majority of criminal offenses against human health is the abstract threat to human health for the fact that the legislator assumes that all the acts of providing medical treatment or other medical assistance done by the persons who do not have the required and adequate professional qualifications create the danger to human health.[350]

---

348 Randelovic, V. op.cit., p.233-248.
349 tojanovic, Z. op.cit., p.818.
350 Stojanovic, Z., Oelic, N. *Krivicno pravo, posebni deo*, Pravni fakuhet Univerzitela u Beogradu, Pravna knjiga, Beograd, 2013, p. 195.

Thus, attempting to prove that medical treatment or provision of medical services have not created danger and have not been harmful to health or even that they have been successful and have helped the recovery of a passive subject is nether relevant nor allowed in the criminal proceedings. According to the stance of the judicial practice, achieving success in medical treatment does not exclude the criminal liability and the existence of the criminal offense of quackery.[351]

The perpetrator of the criminal offense of quackery is the person engaged in treatment without holding a university degree in medicine or dental medicine as well as the person who provides other forms of medical assistance without adequate high school qualifications (medical high school etc.). More precise conditions regarding the required professional qualifications are defined by the Law on Health Care. Thus, the perpetrator may be any person, excluding the persons who have required professional qualifications for providing medical treatment and other medical assistance.[352]

With this incrimination it is essential that the provlslon of medical treatment and medical services should be done without proper professional qualifications, which means that the perpetrator of the criminal offense may be any person without such professional qualifications. That means that the perpetrator may be any person who does not hold a university degree in medicine, but who provides medical treatment or a person without adequate high school qualifications (a high school diploma in medicine), but who provides medical services. Additional conditions in terms of professional qualifications are defined by the Law on Health Care.[353] This leads to the conclusion that only persons who may not be the perpetrators of this criminal offense are those who have the required and adequate professional qualifications.[354] In practice, the perpetrators of the criminal offenses of quackery may be both laymen, i.e. persons who do not have professional knowledge of medical sciences and whose aim is to make financial gain through deception, and self-educated people who acquired their limited knowledge of medical sciences on their own by learning out them from different coursebooks and other sources, but also the persons

351 Supreme Court of Serbia, Department in Novi Sadi, Kz. 589/65, cited according to: Simonovic, D. *Krivicna dela u srpskoj legislativi*, „Sluzbeni glasnik", 2010., p. 521.
352 Stojanovic, z. op.cit., p.818.
353 The Law on Health Care, „*the Official Gazette of the Republic of Serbia*", No. 25. of 3rd April 2019. 354 Stojanovic, Z., Delic, . op.cit., p. 195.

who have vast knowledge of medicine. The latter are usually medical students who have not graduated and who, for instance, needed to pass just a few more exams to complete their university education, but they still did not acquire the university degree in medicine. Examples from practice have shown that these persons have always been good and successful, devoted and careful in practicing medicine, while they have referred more complicated cases to specialist doctors, and thus it has been hard to discover that the persons who practice medicine illegally were in question.[355]

The act of commission of the criminal offense of unlicensed practice of pharmacy (paragraph 2) involves engagement in preparing or issuing medicaments. The criminal offense of unlicensed practice of pharmacy is committed by the person who prepares or issues medications without adequate professional qualifications (Article 254, paragraph 2, of the Criminal Code). Namely, as it is the case with quackery, this criminal offense is committed by a person who does not have prescribed professional qualifications. The perpetrator can be any person who issues or prepares medicaments, while he or she does not have prescribed professional qualifications, i.e. does not have a university degree in pharmacy and does not meet possible additional conditions prescribed by the Law on Medicaments and Medical Devices as well as by bylaws in that area.[356]

With unlicensed practice of pharmacy, like with quackery, the act of comm1ss1on 1s defined alternatively and thus it may involve engagement m preparing or issuing medications. The term *engagement* should be understood in the same way as with the criminal offense of quackery. The object of the criminal offense of unlicensed practice of medicine are medicaments, the definition of which is given in the Law on Medicaments and medical devices.[357] The consequence of unlicensed practice of pharmacy, as it is the case with quackery and the majority of criminal offenses against human health, is the abstract threat to human health.

---

355 Ciric, J., *Nadrilekarsrvo, Pravni Infomator,* No. 9/2006, p. 67.
356 Randelovic, V. op.cit., p.233-248.
357 The Law on Medicaments and Medical Devices, *"the Official Gazelle of the Republic of Serbia",* No.30/2010, 107/20 I 2, I I 3/2017 - other laws adn 105/2017 - another law.

263

It is possible and there are cases in practice that a person without proper professional qualifications prepares or issues medicaments or provides medical treatment without the required professional qualifications. It is arguable whether there is concurrence of this criminal offense with the criminal offense of quackery pursuant to paragraph! of the same Article in that case. Formerly, when these were two separate criminal offenses which, in essence, differed by their legal definitions, there were grounds to assume that there was concurrence. The present solution rather supports the apparent concurrence.[358]

As regards the perpetrator of the criminal offense of unlicensed practice of pharmacy, the question is raised as to whether herbalists may be considered quasi-pharmacists. Herbalists prepare different types of tea, balms and other preparations from various kinds of herbs and plants which they claim to have certain medicinal qualities and help in treating various illnesses, such as migraines, obesity, elevated blood pressure etc. Such preparations are sold in open markets and herbal pharmacies. It often happens that these preparations have not undergone professional inspection, whereas they have been prepared by nonprofessional persons, who do not have a degree in pharmacy. Although some assert that herbalists could be considered quasi-pharmacists in a certain sense, in formal legal terms they are not to be considered as such as they do not prepare medications, but preparations that have certain medicinal qualities.[359] Others contend that the term medicament should be interpreted in a wider sense and that this term should also mean the substances which do not have qualities of a medicament, but are intended for treatment,[360] and thus herbalists could perhaps be considered quasi-pharmacists in that sense.[361]

---

358 Stojanovic, Z. op.cit., p. 819
359 Ciric, J., op.cit., p. 67.
360 Stojanovic, Z., Delic, N. op.cit., p. 195.
36 I Randelovic, V. op.cit., p.233-248.

The object of protection: human health. Both quackery and unlicensed practice of pharmacy may only be committed with premeditation. Certain problems on subjective level could arise in terms of deception (both real and legal) regarding certain alternative means and methods of treatment. In case severe consequences ensue (grave bodily harm or serious impairment of health of a person or the death of a person or several persons), that will constitute qualified forms of quackery and unlicensed practice of pharmacy prescribed by the same provisions of paragraphs 1 and 2 of Article 259.[362] commission of the criminal offense suggests that a collective criminal offense, which is executed in the form of profession, is in question. For the realization of the action of this criminal offense, it is necessary that a perpetrator had acted with readiness to repeat the incriminating actions, while it is not of importance whether he or she performed one or more actions. Quackery is a criminal offense, regardless of the number of cases of treating patients.[363]

Based on the verdict passed by the Fourth Municipal Court in Belgrade, Kz.608/03 of 20.03.2003, the defendant was found guilty for the following reason: "Because she treated the injured party for psoriasis in her beauty salon (she is a beautician by profession) in the following way: Having seen her advertisement in the newspaper, in which she claimed to treat psoriasis, the injured party came to her beauty salon, thinking he was in the doctor's office. On that occasion, in order to treat him, she applied cream to his arms and legs and administered nose drops to him, which she charged 1000 DM, while guaranteeing that the injured party would be successfully cured in 24 hours. Thus, she committed the criminal offense of quackery."[364]

In judicial practice, the question of the relationship between the criminal offense of quackery and unlicensed practice of pharmacy pursuant to Article 254 of the Criminal Code and the criminal offense of fraud pursuant to Article 208 of the Criminal Code has arisen as a matter o debate. For instance,[365] in one case from the judicial practice, the defendant, intending to make illegal

---

362 As the severe consequence which ensues with the majority of the criminal offenses from this chapter is the same, qualified fom1s are defined by the common provisions of Article 259 in order to avoid repetition with all those criminal offense and their fom1s, i.e. for the legislative technique. tojanovic, Z. Kome111ar Krivicnog Zakoniko Republike Srbije, „Sluzbeni glasnik", Belgrade, 2017, p. 827.
363 "Bulletin", Court of Appeal in is, 2019, p. 70.
364 "Verdict" No. Ki. 608/03 of20.03.2003
365 Randelovic, V. op.cit., p.233-248.

265

gain, misled the injured parties by misrepresenting the fact that he was a doctor specialized in surgery who practiced alternative medicine and he kept misleading them by claiming that he would improve their health condition by rendering alternative medical services to them in the form of acupuncture and acupressure, thus making illegal gain, by doing which he committed the continuing criminal offense of fraud pursuant to Article 208, paragraph 1, of the Criminal Code related to Article 61, paragraph 1, of the Criminal Code. The defendant did not have a university degree in medicine and he was a diagnostic medical devices electronics technician, who had graduated from the Faculty of Natural Medicine in Belgrade and had completed various courses in homeopathy, phytotherapy etc. As he worked at the Clinical center in Belgrade as an electronics technician, he altered his pass by adding the prefix Dr before his name, which, according to the statement of the defendant, related to the fact that he was a doctor of natural medicine. Although the court took the stance that this case was the matter of the criminal offense of fraud, there are opinions that although the defendant charged for his medical services, which indicates that his intention was to make illegal gain, the presence of the criminal offense of quackery and unlicensed practice of pharmacy cannot be excluded, considering the fact that the defendant treated the injured parties, thus performing the action of this criminal offense. For that reason, in this case it would be correct to apply the rules on the concurrence of criminal offenses pursuant to Article 60 of the Criminal Code, according to which a defendant has committed several criminal offenses by performing one or more actions which he or she is concurrently tried for.[366] In another case, the court decided that "the perpetrator who had been practicing medicine for a long time without a degree in medicine and received the corresponding income committed the criminal offense of quackery and not the criminal offense of fraud."[367] Whether the case is a matter a criminal offense of quackery of the criminal offense of fraud or the concurrence of these two offenses is a factual question which the courts resolve on a case-to-case basis, taking into consideration the circumstances of the concrete case and the intention of the perpetrator's premeditation.[368]

---

366 For more details, please see: Nenad Jevtic, Da lije nadrilekar samo prevarant, 13ᵗʰ ovember 2018, available at: https://www.pravniportal.com/da-li-je-nadrilekar-samo-prevarant/, accessed in: February 2022.
367 The Supreme Court of Serbia, Kz. 1478/86
368 Randelovic, V. op.cit., p. 233-248.

DETECTION AND PREVENTION OF QUACKERY

After discussing criminal-law aspect of medical malpractice, failure to provide medical assistance and quackery, criminal aspect of quackery as well as legal framework that enables its prevention will be presented in the following text.

Quackery, as an ancient social phenomena, is becoming a popular topic among known experts with the development of modern, scientifically based medicine, when there is a tendency towards complete separation from primitive medicine, which was mainly based on magic powers and superstition. At pre-scientific stage of medicine, treatment was performed in the manners in which poisonous substances were eliminated from the body, while treatment of psychological disorders involved exorcism of evil spirits, and, in those times, quackery was in bloom, while in some countries it was even legally regulated as a legal type of craft. With the development of modern medicine and emergence of a large number of professionally trained doctors, a battle for prevention of quackery, as a harmful and a dangerous phenomenon, begins. In the laws of other countries, quackery is prescribed by law as a criminal offense because it poses abstract danger to human health.[369]

When criminal offense of quackery is in question, it is very important to detect it and explain it, as it requires a systematic and thorough approach because of its specificity. In relation to this, it is necessary to take all operational and tactical, technical and evidentiary measures and actions in order to explain the above mentioned criminal offense and discover its perpetrator.

Prevention and detection of a wide range of manifestations of the criminal offense of quackery, and, even more, its proving is increasingly the result of joint and coordinated work of different state and other bodies and organizations (police, public prosecutor's offices, health inspection etc.), while everyone within their jurisdiction use the powers they dispose of to contribute to this goal.

---

369 Ibidem.

Suppression of crime is one of the police activities, whose main function is to prevent, detect and apprehend the perpetrator of a criminal offense and bring them to the competent authority. Prevention and suppression (repression) of crime, i.e. police actions before and after the crime, pervade the entire work of the police. Police activities on prevention and suppression of crime have had decisive influence on the separation of the operational work from other activities in police practice in a certain way for being direct, concrete and linked with other police activities. Operational work[370], in broader sense, involves work on the execution of practical police tasks, i.e. the work of operational police officers, operatives, who perform security tasks in practice, involves, above all, the prevention and suppression of crime.[371]

Operational work of the police is carried out during preliminary investigation proceedings[372] either upon the police's own initiative or at the request of public prosecutor, with the aim of gathering evidence and information for launching criminal proceedings, but also with the aim of preventing the commission of a criminal offense. Operational work may be also defined as a set of criminal and operational methods and means applied and actions taken in accordance with the principle of confidentiality, with the aim of gathering evidence and information which indicate that there is suspicion that a criminal offense has been committed or is planned to be committed, as well as suspicion that a person has committed a criminal offense. The aim of this form of action is to enable the provision of evidence, detecting and solving of a crime, finding and apprehending the perpetrators and bring them to competent authorities, with measures and action taken by the police and other state bodies. Prevention is characterized by identifiability, and repression is characterized by the identification of torts.[373]

---

370 Operational work (lat. *operari* = operate, work) is composed of the following by its content: 1) taking measures for the purpose of detection of criminal offenses, discovering and fixing the traces and object of criminal offenses, and 2) taking measures for the purpose of perpetrators of criminal offenses and preventing their escape or hiding ad well as their discovery and apprehending.

371 Miletic, S. i Jugovic., S., *Pravo unutrasnjih poslova,* KPA, Beograd, 2009., p. 215.

372 Criminal proceedings are composed of: preliminary proceedings (preliminary investigation proceedings, an investigation and an indicting procedure), main proceedings (the preparation of the main hearing, the main hearing and the pronouncing and proclaiming of the first-instance judgment) and ordinary and extraordinary legal remedy proceedings. Preliminary investigation proceedings precede an investigation. Preliminary investigation proceedings are conducted for the grounded suspicion that a criminal offense which is prosecuted *ex officio* has been committed. A public prosecutor is in charge of preliminary investigation proceedings, while all this stage the police acts upon the requests/orders from the public prosecutor.

373 For more information, please see: Zarkovic, M. i dr. *Kriminalistika,* VSUP, Beograd, 1997., p. 23-24.

Operational police work on suppression and prevention of quackery as well as crime on the whole must be organized and systematic, involving mutual cooperation with a public prosecutor, above all, as well as with a person in charge of preliminary investigation and other bodies and institutions, most importantly health inspection and other inspection bodies, in terms of suppression of illegal, unlawful activities in the field of medical treatments and providing other medical services. The police indirectly participates in detecting this criminal offense, collecting personal and material evidence[374] through the application of appropriate operational measures and actions.

According to the valid legal provisions, detection, suppression and prevention of this kind of criminal offenses is the area of activity of police officers of the criminal police and this type of criminal offenses is within the competence of the police officers who prevent and suppress financial crime. Police officers perform police work by using their powers and taking measures and action in accordance with the Law on Police, Criminal Procedure Code and other laws and bylaws, while adhering to the principles of legality, confidentiality, truthfulness, objectivity, efficiency and rationality in work, protection of source and intelligence as well as to other tenets and principles of criminology.

Successful detection of a criminal offense of quackery also involves the constant monitoring of the manifested modi operandi in the commission of this criminal offense in practice as well as adequate analysis of the manifestations of this criminal offense. In that way, the initial basis for observing certain modi operandi in quackery is created, which enables timely planning of operational activities aimed at solving and proving this criminal offense. The creation of the initial basis or indications[375] which point to the grounds to suspect that this criminal offence has been committed should be the result of work of all competent authorities for suppression of quackery.

---

374 Personal evidence represents the facts the source of which is a man who has directly observed them with his or her senses or indirectly learnt about them, while material evidence are facts the source of which are written documents, personal documents, objects and items in a certain connection with the criminal act.

375 The term "indication" (Latin indici11111, meaning sign) is often used in everyday speech to denote certain phenomena in reality which give cause for suspicion of existence or nonexistence of a certain "thing" (a fact, circumstances, a situation, an event, ...). In accordance with that, in criminal terminology, indications denote certain facts or circumstances which point indirectly to the existence of a criminal offense or to its perpetrator and other important elements of significance for taking action in a concrete criminal matter. For more information, please see: Zarkovic, M. Kriminalisticka taktika, Kriminalisticko-policijska akademija, Belgrade, 20 I 4, p. 44.

According to the provisions of the Criminal Procedure Code of the Republic of Serbia, state and other authorities, legal entities and natural persons report criminal offenses which are prosecuted ex officio, and which they have been informed of or learnt about in another way, under the circumstance foreseen by law or other regulations.[376] They file a criminal charge[377] to the competent prosecutor's office or to the police, which is responsible for receiving the criminal charge and forwarding it to the public prosecutor for further handling and decision on the basis of the mentioned code.

Preliminary investigation procedure starts with learning about the founded suspicion that a criminal offense for which the perpetrator is prosecuted *ex officio* has been committed. Greater part of the criminal police activity takes place at this stage and it mainly involves taking informal measures and action (operational and tactical measures and action) and exceptionally evidentiary measures. From the aspect of the type of action taken in the process of detecting criminal offenses and their perpetrators, the priority is given to informal, i.e. operational and tactical measures and action, which is in line with the fundamental function and the essential task of the authorities of the Ministry of the Interior, and that is detection of criminal offenses and perpetrators.[378]

Apart from the authority to conduct an investigation, a public prosecutor has the authority to manage a preliminary investigation in which the police takes action. The aim of public prosecutor in a preliminary investigation is to work in cooperation with the police to collect evidence which indicate that there is a link between a criminal offense and a perpetrator and thus enable further criminal proceedings or to prevent launching of criminal proceedings when there are no grounds for doing so.

---

376 Criminal Procedure Code "the Official Gazette of the Republic of Serbia", No. 72/201 I, l01/201 I, 121/2012, 32/2013, 45/2013, 55/2014, 35/2019, 27/202 I - decision made by the Supreme Court 162/2021 - decision made by the Supreme Court)
377 A criminal charge is a written or oral statement made to the competent authority about a potentially committed criminal offense and a potential perpetrator. A criminal charge can be defined as a written or oral document by which the public prosecutor is informed of the commission of a criminal offense which is prosecuted *ex officio* or that there arc grounds to suspect or facts which indicate that it has been committed. The form of a criminal charge is not defined nor is the mandatory content.
378 Bejatovic, S. i B. Banovic. *Radnje organa unutrasnjih poslova u pretkrivicnom i prethodnom krivicnom postupku i njihova dokazna vrednost;* in: Zbomik radova Polozaj i uloga policije u pretkrivicnom i prethodnom krivicnom postupku, Belgrade: Visa skola unutrasnjih poslova, 2004, p. l 7-32.

A public prosecutor as an authority managing the preliminary investigation has several possibilities at his or her disposal if he or she is unable to assess whether what is mentioned in a criminal charge is probable or if the information in the criminal charge do not offer sufficient grounds to make decision whether an investigation would be conducted. Firstly, he or she may gather the necessary information, summon citizens for the purpose of collecting the necessary information, following the same procedure used by the police authorities, or he or she may submit a request to public or other authorities and legal entities to provide necessary information. If a public prosecutor is unable to take action on his or her own, he or she may request the police to collect the necessary information and to take other measures and action with a view to detecting a criminal offense and a perpetrator. The police is obliged to take action upon the request from a public prosecutor and to inform him or her of the measures and action it has taken within 30 days from the day it received the request.

If there are grounds to suspect that a criminal offense which is prosecuted *ex officio* has been committed, the police is obliged to take necessary measures so as to find the perpetrator of the criminal offense, so that the perpetrator or an accomplice would not hide or escape, so as to discover and secure the traces of the criminal offense and the objects which may serve as evidence as well as to collect all the information which could be of use for the successful conducting of the criminal proceedings. In order to fulfill the mentioned duties, the police can: collect the necessary information from citizens, conduct the necessary control of means of transport, passengers and luggage, restrict the movement at certain space for the required period of time, which may not exceed eight hours, take necessary measures in relation to the identification of persons and objects, issue a search for a person or objects that are wanted, search certain facilities and premises of the state authorities, companies, stores and other legal entities in the presence of a responsible person, examine their documents and seize it, if necessary, and take other necessary measures and action. Upon the order of a judge for preliminary proceedings, based on the proposal of a public prosecutor, the police may obtain records of communication made by telephone, used cell towers and locate the place from which the communication was made in order to fulfill its duties in accordance with the Criminal Procedure

Code. It is obliged to inform a public prosecutor of measures and action taken without delay and not later than 24 hours after they were taken.

With the criminal offense of quackery, the essential and most important source of information about its commission is the person injured by quackery. Apart from the injured party, the source of information about committed quackery may be the reports made by citizens (injured parties), possible witnesses, if the injured party does not report the offense for certain reasons, anonymous reports, direct (street, patrol and operational) police activity. Moreover, other sources of information, which are not less important, are also the mass media, the internet, social networks, various other media, professional associations, health inspection, speaking in public etc.

As a result of the lack of knowledge or education, the majority of citizens who visit a doctor to be provided with a required medical service rendered by a doctor or other health care workers do not use the Registers of the competent chambers in order to check whether a doctor has a work license or not, whether he or she is entered in a chamber's register or not nor do they use the register of the Business Registers Agency (BRA). By searching the information on the website of the BRA available on the internet, a citizen may obtain information on: whether a doctor's office/a health-service institution/ a clinic is entered in the register of the BRA, and if it is, when, the data on the head office, the responsible person, the founders, the date of foundation and registration, business activity, the amount of capital, the bank accounts numbers, published founding acts and documents on the status etc. Thus, before visiting a doctor's office/a health-service institution/ a clinic for receiving treatment and/or being rendered other medical services, a citizen may search the register of the BRA in order to check whether that facility is registered as a doctor's office, may check the license on the website of the Serbian Medical Chamber, may see whether there is a work license visibly displayed in the office, together with the decision issued by the BRA and the labor inspection license. A citizen may check whether a certain prescribed/recommended substance or medication is in the National Register of Medicines of the Medicines and Medical Devices Agency. It is very important that a citizen makes a thorough check where he or she is going and who he or she visits prior to any medical services, treatments and procedures. A citizen can check information on a doctor's office and a doctor he or she is interested in very quickly by directly accessing the internet website of the Serbian Medical Chamber (which can give information on whether a doctor has a work license or whether he or she works without it), while the website of the BRA can give important information on the health care providers (whether a doctor's office is entered in the Register, and if it is, when, the data on its head office, the responsible person etc.).

In case of deterioration of the health condition, it is necessary that a citizen should address a competent physician of the health-service institution (a health center etc.). If there is any suspicion that a citizen has been rendered a medical service by a person without adequate professional qualifications, i.e. that quackery is in question, it is necessary that he or she should address and report the case to the competent authority (a public prosecutor's office, the police, the health inspection etc.). It is the very lack of information and knowledge that are the important reasons for which quack doctors often go unpunished so a citizen should never hesitate if he or she has been a victim of or a witness to this criminal offense as there are competent authorities he or she can address.

Practice has shown that citizens learn about and come to quack doctors, the persons who misrepresent themselves as doctors in public and on social networks, usually through advertisements on the Instagram and Facebook social networks, or by being recommended by acquaintances and friends who have allegedly been satisfied with the medical services provided. Quack doctors who perform aesthetic procedures (mesotherapy, botox and hyaluronic acid injections, chemical peeling etc.) which can only be performed in health-service institutions and in private practice founded as a general and specialist MD's or DMD's office or a polyclinic and which can only be performed by MDs or DMDs, as it is foreseen by the Professional Methodology Instructions for Practicing Anti-aging Medicine of the Ministry of Health[379] (i.e. only

---

379 The Professional Methodology Instructions for Practicing Anti-aging Medicine define specific conditions, methods and procedures for practicing anti-aging medicine in a health-service institution and private practice as well as conditions which the lecturers in programs of continuing education must meet and other important issues, by which the conditions for obtaining a work licence for anti-aging medicine are satisfied. (*Strucno merodolosko uputstvo za obavljanje metoda „anriejdz." medicine* No. 500-01- 1246/2018-2 of I 9.09.2018)

professionally qualified doctors with a license may perform aesthetic surgery procedures), also advertise procedures performed on patients on their web pages, even though they do not have adequate professional qualifications, i.e. they are not doctors of medicine or doctors of dental medicine, and they perform the procedures on the premises which do not meet the required conditions for work, using medical devices and material (of dubious origin and quality) which have not been authorized by the Medicines Agency. do not have adequate professional qualifications, i.e. they are not doctors of medicine or doctors of dental medicine, and they perform the procedures on the premises which do not meet the required conditions for work, using medical devices and material (of dubious origin and quality) which have not been authorized by the Medicines Agency.

The head office of unregistered doctor's offices is most usually in rented beauty salons, in apartments and facilities. Quack doctors often hire real doctors and other medical staff (general practitioners, specialist doctors, surgeons, nurses, anesthesiologists), who are unaware of being hired by a quack doctor. They learn about the fact that they have been working with a quack doctor only after he or she is prosecuted. Doctors are motivated by fee to be hired by a quack doctor. These medical procedures are in high demand and are very expensive, especially when plastic and reconstructive surgery is in question. Incidentally, the communication between a patient and a quack doctor can be established and take place via a cell phone, social networks, Viber, WhatsApp and other mobile applications, where the appointment, place and time of a medical procedure and the fee are arranged precisely.

Not suspecting a quack doctor, a patient goes to the agreed place, where he or she is subjected to a medical procedure. After providing a medical service, a quack doctor usually issues a patient with a medical reports and results with his or her signature, so as not to be suspected, and verified with a forged signature stamp and office stamp. In order to hide their illegal activities, quack doctors issue a patient with false test results allegedly produced by a reference laboratory, e.g. a histopathology report, thus misleading the patient into thinking that his or her sample has been sent and that everything is fine with it, while the reality is completely different, which may have serious consequences for the health and life of the patient. Not suspecting the authenticity of the medical report and prescribed therapy, the patient adheres to the instructions given by

274

the quack doctor. It is only when discomfort appears that he or she endeavors to re-establish communication with the quack doctor to have the discomfort relieved or the injury treated. However, it is then that the problem arises because the communication with the quack doctor fails to be established, and the patient realizes he or she was misled into thinking he or she had visited a doctor and it becomes clear to him or her that he or she was deceived. When they are discovered and when they start receiving the complaints from patients, quack doctors tend to get rid of and destroy objects and traces of the criminal offense.

The first piece of information that a criminal offense has been committed is usually received within the report submitted by an injured person. This is mainly the information on persons who suffered bodily harm or considerable health damage from the treatment given by quack doctors. Apart from the injured parties, the reports from possible witnesses and citizens acquainted with the case appear as the source of information when an injured party does not report the offense for certain reasons. Moreover, such information may be published on social networks and internet portals of various media. All these ways of learning about the cases represent a significant source of information for the criminal police and the competent prosecutor's office as well as grounds to suspect that certain persons have committed criminal offenses which are prosecuted ex officio. The competent public prosecutor submits the request the request for gathering the required information and taking other measures and action to the police for the purpose of detecting the criminal offense and discovering the perpetrator and the police is obliged to act upon this request.

After receiving the request for gathering necessary information from the competent prosecutor's office, the criminal police starts its work, primarily by drafting the plan of operational action and conducting checks. What follows is the work on the recognition and identification of the suspects on the basis of the photographs of potential perpetrators of the criminal offense published by the injured parties, by looking through the photo album of the perpetrators of criminal offenses, checks through the records of the Ministry of the Interior and other state authorities, organizations and institutions etc. Following that, the injured parties are identified on the basis of the checks through operational records of persons (administrative affairs), field checks and interviews with the responsible persons of the mass media and internet portals which are conducted so as to establish the identity of injured persons as well as the address of their permanent or temporary residence.

After the injured persons are identified, the criminal police conducts interviews[380] with them in their capacity as citizens on the official premises. A detailed interview should be conducted with injured parties[381] regarding all the circumstances of a criminal offense, while care should be taken of the special psychophysical state an injured party is in. The aim of the interview with an injured party is to obtain detailed information on the perpetrators of criminal offenses, ways in which they found out about the quack doctors and the place of commission, to identify potential witnesses, employees (doctors, nurses and technicians), to obtain information on the job description, actions they performed, the amount of the fees charged as well as to seize medical reports and other documents from the injured parties for the purpose of forensic analysis. An injured party should give the police a detailed personal description as much as that is possible, while it should not be insisted on details or at least not during the first interview. An injured party should also provide the information on distinctive features and speech characteristics of perpetrators so that the injured party could identify them, on which occasion he or she is presented with the photo album of registered perpetrators for indirect identification or at least for pointing to the similarities of the personal description of perpetrators to the ones which are to be found in the photo album.

---

380 Terminologically, in conducting interviews with victims, witnesses and suspects, the following expression are used as synonyms in professional literature: forensic interview, gathering of information, examination, informative interview, interrogation, statement, collecting of information.

381 The term "an injured party" is present in criminal and criminological terminology as well as in the provisions of the national criminal legislation. In this connection, only the valid procedural legislation defines the meaning of the term "an injured party", where it is used to denote a person who e personal or property right has been violated or jeopardized by a criminal offense; (Criminal Procedure Law). In comparison to the Criminal Procedure Code, which docs not recognize the term "a victim" at all, but recognizes only an injured party in different procedural situations and roles, the Criminal Code uses the expression "an injured party" as well as the term "a victim" of a criminal offense. An injured party and a victim are recognized as passive subjects of a criminal offense, i.e. as persons injured or damaged by a criminal offense. In that connection, a victi1n is person on or against whom an act of commission of a criminal offense was done, while an injured party is the bearer (holder) of goods that are protected and injured or damaged by a criminal offense (apart from a physical person, the injured party may also be a legal entity). For more details, please see: Zarkovic, M., *Kriminalisricka taktika*, Kriminalisticko-policijska akademija, Belgrade, 2014, p. 135-136.

Furthermore, an interview will be conducted with all the persons who may be acquainted with certain relevant facts in relation to the concrete criminal offense and its perpetrator, i.e. who may have information of relevance for the detection of a criminal offense and its perpetrator. In that sense, apart from the persons injured as result of a criminal offense, the providers of information may also be witnesses, experts and the like. In each individual case, the operational activity should be directed to gathering material and personal evidence as the combination of them is the best way to prove criminal offenses.

The criminal police applies its legal powers which are defined m Article 286, paragraph 2, of the Criminal Procedure Code, in cooperation and coordination with the competent public prosecutor, and they represent checks conducted at accredited educational academic and professional institutions in the area of medical sciences and high schools of medicine so as to establish whether the perpetrators who have practiced quackery, i.e. the persons suspected of providing treatments and/or other medical services without adequate professional qualifications possibly have adequate professional qualifications for this activity or not with the aim of proving the substance of the criminal offense of quackery.

Alongside this, checks are conducted at the Business Registers Agency of the Republic of Serbia, on which occasion the criminal police gathers evidence on whether the persons who practiced quackery had a registered office, institution, institute or clinic at all and if they did, when they had it and whether it was registered in their name or in the name of their relatives and friends.

The Ministry of Health of the Republic of Serbia necessarily obtains evidence as to whether the persons suspected of quackery possessed the required - necessary work licenses, whereas the health inspection gathers data on whether those persons have been a subject of inspection, and when and which time period they were the subject of control, whether and which measures were taken against the responsible persons if it is established that they have been the subject of inspection.

The evidence on the employment status of the suspects, i.e. years of service, place of employment and the amount of income and contributions are obtained from the Pension and Disability Insurance Fund of the Republic of Serbia, while the criminal police may also collect similar evidence in the Central Register of Mandatory Social Security Insurance.

The operational field work of the criminal police involves taking operational action in the form of checks conducted at health care workers chambers (the Serbian Medical Chamber, the Serbian Dental Chamber, the Pharmaceutical Chamber of Serbia, the Serbian Chamber of Biochemists, the Chamber of Nurses and Health Care Technicians of Serbia) with a view to obtaining evidence as to whether quack doctors have possibly been entered in the Register of these chambers and what period they were entered in it, whether they possess the work license, which specialization in the area of medical sciences they have been issued with the license for, whether their license has been revoked, why their license was revoked and which decision was the revocation based on, whether and when they were deleted from the register, whether the measure of the termination of the performance of medical activity has been imposed and for how long.

If the information is obtained that a person who practiced quackery hired medical staff, then what follows is the identification of the staff members. In addition to this, the criminal police takes criminal measures and action in relation to the medical staff, which are directed at obtaining evidence such as: employment contract in the health-service institutions where the staff members are actually employed with permits, licenses and diplomas in acquired education and certificates of professional qualifications from the personnel files. Following that, the required information is gathered from the medical staff who are interviewed in their capacity as citizens on the circumstances of their engagement which a quack doctor they were hired by, whether they concluded a contract regulating additional or supplementary work, where and in which exact place they worked, their job descriptions, how their fees were paid, directly or in the account, in advance or following the performed medical procedure or surgery, how much they were paid, what currency they were paid in, whether these payment operations were recorded in the business records and in fiscal cash registers, and if not, whether the receipts on the payments made were issued, how the patients were treated, which devices and medications were used, who defined the therapy or whether all the actions and the activities were performed illegally (known as illegal employment). Depending on the roles and activities of medical staff and collected material evidence, the competent public prosecutor may grant these persons a status of a witness or an accessory and an accomplice in the criminal offense during the preliminary investigation and in the course of further criminal proceedings.

The criminal police in charge of detecting this kind of criminal offenses conducts searches of apartments, premises and persons based on the court order (evidentiary action foreseen by the Criminal Procedure Code) with the aim of discovering and finding the perpetrator of a criminal offense, finding objects and traces of a criminal offense and their securing. If an object or objects of a criminal offense are found during the search, the objects and documents are provisionally seized and they are taken away, kept and stored duly for further forensic analysis and examination which will be done in the criminal proceedings. The criminal police issues a certificate of provisionally seized objects in relation to the confiscation of objects. The competent public prosecutor is informed thereof and consulted regarding the necessary measures and action to be taken.

It very important to outline that when a doctor's office, a room or a facility where a criminal offense was committed is discovered, when objects and traces of a criminal offense are discovered, the notification of that is given to the competent public prosecutor and the Department for Crime Scene Investigation, which will take photographs and video recordings of that, secure and, if necessary, provisionally seize the objects and traces of criminal offense for further forensic examination. Based on the court order, the competent public prosecutor in the preliminary investigation procedure may request the criminal police to conduct a crime scene investigation and the forensic examination of discovered items and documents, mobile telephones and computers so that its contents, the actual owner, telephone communication made and correspondence via text messages would be established. The criminal police is assisted in detecting and solving this kind of criminal offenses by the National Center for Criminal Forensics, which conducts the entire necessary forensic examination. When all evidence and traces are gathered, the qualification of the criminal offense is determined in cooperation with a public prosecutor and further action is taken to discover and arrest the perpetrator of the criminal offense. Perpetrators of this kind of criminal offenses may have their financial situation checked prior to or in the course of the criminal proceedings at the the request of the competent public prosecutor as a form of financial investigation conducted in cooperation with other state authorities.

In order to find and arrest perpetrators of the criminal offense of quackery, the criminal police drafts an operational plan. The criminal police is supported in the implementation of this legal power by other police units. The police is authorized to issue a search for a person or for objects in order to find and arrest perpetrators of this kind of criminal offenses and prevent a person from escaping in accordance with the provisions of the Criminal Procedure Code. This authority may be used for the purpose of prevention when it is not possible to establish the place of permanent or temporary residence of a perpetrator of a criminal offense or his or her whereabouts. Moreover, if the need arises, the police initiates special evidentiary actions, which are subject to approval from competent public prosecutor's office, and informs of the results of the application of the approved measure. It drafts the request for the provision of records of communication made by telephone, used cell towers and locations from which the communication was made in cooperation with the competent prosecutor with a view to discovering perpetrators of criminal offenses.

The criminal work on detection and solving this kind of criminal offenses requires the police to act timely and efficiently as otherwise the objects and traces of a criminal offense may be destroyed and the perpetrator of the criminal offense may escape or hide. In all stages of criminal police action, one of the most important principles is the principle of lawful acting and respecting the rules of the profession.

After all checks have been completed by the criminal police and upon prior consultations with the competent prosecutor, further action is taken to arrest the perpetrator of the criminal offense. The discovery of the suspect enables direct identification by both the injured party(ies) and possible witnesses. Authorized by the competent public prosecutor and in accordance with the law, the police orders 48-hour detention to the suspect, who will be brought before the competent prosecutor's office with the criminal charge and evidence.

The text that follows presents the examples (cases) of quackery m practice:

On 24th May 2021, the officers of the Ministry of the Interior in Belgrade arrested S.K. (1998) and D.K. (1972) from Belgrade for founded suspicion that they committed the criminal offense of unauthorized engagement in a certain activity, grave offense against human health, quackery and unlicensed practice of pharmacy. S.K. is charged with providing medical services and performing medical procedures on patients for a fee from January last year to April this year, without the required professional qualifications, concealing the fact that he had not been professionally trained. After performing medical procedures, he issued medical reports with the prescribed medications to the injured patients. This resulted in the grave impairment of the injured patients' health. His mother D.K assisted him with premeditation in doing this.

The suspects were ordered 48 hours' detention and they will be brought before the competent prosecutor's office with the criminal charge.[382]

On 1st June 2021, the officers of the Ministry of the Interior in Belgrade arrested O. M. (1990) for there were grounds to suspect that she had committed the criminal offenses of unauthorized engagement in a certain activity, grave offenses against human health and quackery and unlicensed practice of pharmacy. She is charged with providing aesthetic medical services to patients for a fee from April 2020 to 15th March 2021, in an unregistered aesthetic studio in the territory of the municipality of Savski Venac, without the required professional qualifications and without the required approval for independent work, for the performance of which she is required by law to have the permit issued by the competent authority. Concealing the fact that she was not professionally trained for providing medical services and performing medical procedures, O. M., as it is suspected, did not issue medical reports, fiscal or other receipts to the patients following the procedures, but she prescribed them medications orally, which resulted in the grave impairment of the health of injured parties, i.e. patients.

---

382 The announcement of the Ministry of the Interior of Serbia available at: http://www.mup. gov.rs/wps/portal/sr/aktuelno/saopstenja/d5d6e2c3-7640-4715-97b0-2e4dbdd892cb, visited on: 14.02.2022.

The suspect was ordered 48-hour detention and she will be brought before the First Principal Public Prosecutor's Office in Belgrade with the criminal charge.[383]

On 20th October 2021, the officers of the Ministry of the Interior in Belgrade arrested O. L. (197 4) for there were grounds to suspect that she had committed the criminal offenses of unauthorized engagement in a certain activity and quackery and unlicensed practice of pharmacy. It it suspected that at the start of August last year she provided aesthetic medical services to an injured party in an unregistered facility in New Belgrade, without the required professional qualifications and a MD and DMD license. The suspect was ordered 48-hour detention and she will be brought before the Third Principal Public Prosecutor's Office with the criminal charge.[384]

383 The announcement of the Ministry of the Interior of Serbia available al: http://www.mup.gov.rs/wps/portal/sr/aktuelno/saopslenja/d5d6e2c3-7640-4715-97b0-2e4dbdd892cb,visited on: 14. 02. 2022
384 The announcement of the Ministry of the Interior of Serbia available at: http://www. mup.gov.rs/wps/porta 1/sr/aktuel no/saopsten ja/d5d6e2c3-7640-4 715-97 b0-2e4dbdd892c b, visited on: 14. 02. 2022.

BIOGRAPHIES

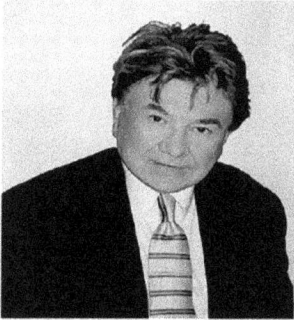

Dr. Borko Dordevic, PhD in Medicine, graduated from the Fifth Grammar School in 1961. He gained a degree in medicine at the University of Belgrade School of Medicine in 1968.

Dr. Dordevic has lived in the USA since 1971, where the degree he was awarded by the the University of Belgrade School of Medicine was validated. There, he continued his specialization in general and plastic surgery, which he completed in 1977, thus earning the title of specialist in plastic and reconstructive surgery, surgery of the hand and genitalia, maxillofacial and aesthetic surgery. At the start of 1978 he opened a private practice in Palm Springs and Beverly Hills, California. He worked there until 1989 and from that time he practiced only aesthetic surgery. At the same time, Dr. Dordevic opened the Mediterranean Surgery Center for Plastic and Reconstructive Surgery in Igalo, Montenegro, in cooperation with the *Dr. Sima Milosevic* Institute.

In 1994 he received a PhD degree at the Belgrade University with the thesis on secondary rhinoplasty and he was awarded the title of Doctor of Medical Sciences. In September 1996 Dr. Dordevic was awarded the title of Associate Professor of Plastic and Reconstructive Surgery at the Belgrade University School of Medicine, and in March he was awarded the same title at the University of Nis School of Medicine.

In the USA he gained the following certifications: ECFMG, FLEX, the American Board of Plastic and Reconstructive Surgery certificate, the Advanced Trauma Life Support certificate and the American Board of Cosmetic Surgery certificate. He is the member of numerous professional organizations abroad, such as: American Medical Association, American College of Emergency Physicians, Royal Academy of Medicine, New York Academy of Sciences, Palm Springs Academy of Medicine, American Society of Outpatient Surgeons, International College Surgeons, American Academy of Aesthetic and Restorative Surgery, American Academy of Cosmetic

Surgery, American Society of Liposuction Surgery, The Skin Laser Center of New Jersey.

He is the author of many publications in the area of plastic and reconstructive surgery in Serbia and abroad, and his ten-volume Coursebook on Plastic, Reconstructive and Aesthetic Surgery, published by Atlanta International Ltd, Belgrade, is presently in print.

After decades-long outstanding practice in the USA, Professor Dordevic shares his unrivaled and vast knowledge with the young generation, future doctors and health care workers here in Serbia as well. He is the author of the set of five coursebooks on reconstructive and plastic surgery, which are more that significant for the education of medical experts in this area.

What first-class plastic surgeon Dr. Dordevic is is best illustrated by the BBC, which places him among the top ten plastic surgeons in the world ever. His work is the best reflection of that. It is not by accident that he has been requested to create Saddam Hussein look-alikes. Apart from that, he also created the look-alikes of Elvis Presley as well as of many other world stars such as Larry King, Sir Elton John, Joan Collins, Gabor sisters and other celebrities in the world of sports and public figures.

In 2010 Professor Dordevic received yet another prestigious award -Ellis Island Medal of Honor. This award is presented annually to 100 most eminent people in the world in their professional and humanitarian work, who, among others, include four Presidents of the United States.

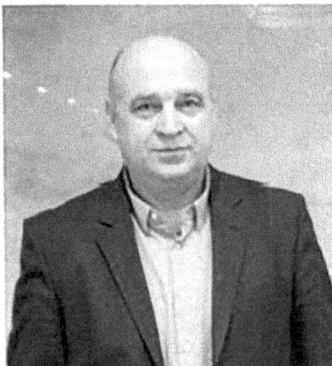

Dr. Dragan Cvetkovic was born 25th September 1967 in Gnjilane, the Repiblic of Serbia. He is employed with the Ministry of the Interior of the Republic of Serbia, where he works on the combating financial crime. Along his professional engagement, he has continued his advanced education and research and scientific work, in the course of which he has gained academic and scientific titles.

He holds a PhD degree in Economics, and he is an MA and specialist in Criminology as well as a certified forensic accountant. He is a highly qualified expert with years-long experience and theoretical knowledge in the area of prevention and detection of all forms of financial crime. He is also the member of the Association of Certified Fraud Examiners (ACFA). He is a Visiting Lecturer at the University of Criminal Investigation and Police Studies as well as the Faculty of Organizational Sciences of the University of Belgrade. Over the past years, he was the lecturer of courses intended for criminal investigators organized by the Ministry of the Interior of the Republic of Serbia.

As a lecturer, he participated in the course on "Professional Training for Investigators of Misuse and Fraudulent Acts in the Area of Economic and Financial Forensics" organized by the Republic Institute for Forensic Expertise (*Republicki zavod za sudska vestacenja A.D.*) in Novi Sad at the Faculty of Organizational Sciences. He participated on several occasions in the organization of the seminar on "the Protection in Corporate Sector from Fraudulent Acts in Financial Reports" in his capacity as a practical expert at the Faculty of Organizational Sciences.

Moreover, he participated as a lecturer in the seminar on "Prevention of Misuse in Public Tenders - the practice of the Prosecutor's Offices and the Ministry of the Interior", organised by CMN and the National Center for Corporate Education. He is also a lecturer in courses on "Forensics in Practice - Legal-Economic, Security and Information Aspect", organized by the Belgrade Business and Arts Academy of Applied Studies.

He is the author and co-author of numerous handbooks, publications and articles in the area of forensic accounting, financial criminology, financial crime, money laundering and other.

He is married to Snezana, a doctor subspecialist in pulmology, with whom he has a daughter Jelena (1999) and a son Marko (2002). He lives with his family in Belgrade.

REFERENCES

Albrecht, W. Steven., Albrecht , Chad. Fraud *Examination&-Prevention,*Thomson-South-Western, Ohio, 2004.

Altamura C. Paluello MD, Clinical and subclinical body dismorphic disorder, Eur Arch Psychiatry Clinic neuroscience, 2001.

Alton WG Jr. *Malpractice: a trial lawyer's advice for physicians.* Boston: Little, Brown, 1977.

Anders G. *More insurers pay for care that's in trials.* Wall St. Journal, 15ᵗʰ February, 1994.

Annot., 37 A.L.R.2d 464 (1971, Supp. 1984).

Argyris, C. *Integrating the individual and organization.* New York, Wiley, 1964.

Aubert v. Hospital "Charity", 363 Co.2nd 1223 (La. App. 1978.) *Avoiding managed care's liability risks.* Med Econ, 25th April, 1994 Ayala, A., i dr., Ljudska prava u zdravstvenoj zastiti: prirucnik za prakticare, Medicinski fakultet Univerziteta u Beogradu, 2015.

Ask the Experts. Insurance Corporation, of American Malpratice

Report, May, 1992.

A costly lesson in lab-testfollow-up. Med Econ, 25th April, 1994. Azevedo D. *Courts let UR firms off the hook-and leave doctors on.*

Med Econ, 25ᵗʰ January, 1993.

Banovic, J. *Ultima ratio karakter krivicnog prava u svetlu krivicnog dela Gradenje bez gradevinske dozvole (cl. 219a KZ).* Crimen (Beograd), 10(1), 2019., p. 69-86. available at: https://doi. org/10.5937 /crimen 1901069B

Baldasare v. Suriano, 175 AD.2nd 93,571 N.Y.S.2nd 797 (1991.)

Bartlett E. and Rehmar, M. *The difficult patient.* Baltimor, EBA, Associates.

Bejatovic, S. i B. Banovic. *Radje organa unutrasnjih poslova u pretkrivicnom i prethodnom krivicnom postupku i njihova dokazna vrednost;* u: Zbornik radova Polozaj i uloga policije u pretkrivicnom i prethodnom krivicnom postupku, Beograd: Visa skola unutrasnjih poslova, 2004., p. 17-32.

Bell v. Umstattd, 401 S. W.2nd 306 (Tex. Civ App. 1966,.

Berglund S . *To see ourselves as other see us.* The Pulse, American Physicians Exchange, May, 1992.

"Bilten", Apelacioni sud u Nisu, 2019.

Blake, R. and Mouton, JS. *The managerial grid.* Hjuston, Gulf Publishing, 1964.

Borne v. Brumfield, 363 So. 2nd 79, 83 (La. App. 1978.)

Barak J, Veilleux S. Informed consent in emergency settings. *Ann Emerg Med* 1984;

Caldwell vs Overton, 554 S.W.2nd 832

Campion FX. *Grand Rounds on Medical Malpractice.* Chicago, American Medical Association, 1991.

Caesar NB. *How to gain leverage with a health plan.* Med Econ, 7th February, 1994.

Cezeaux v. Libby, 539 S.W.2nd 187 (Tex. Civ. App. 1976.) Chittenden WA. *Malpractice liability and managed health care: history and prognosis.* Torts and Ins Law J, Vol. 26, No. 3, 451-496, spring, 1991.

Coleman v. California Friends Chuck, 81 P 2d 469, 470, Cal 1938; *Schneider v. Little Company,* 151 NW, 588, Mich 1915; Pike v. Honsinger, 49 NE 760, NY 1898; "The Standard of Care, Parts I, II, and III," 225 *JAMA* No. 6, page 671, August 3, 1973; 225 *JAMA* No. 7, page 791, August 13, 1973, 225 *JAMA* Mo. 8, page 1027, August 20, 1973; *Adkins v. Ropp,* 14 NE 2d 727, Ind 1938.

Courts support health insurers that reject "unnecessary" care. Wall St. Journal, 25th November, 1992.

Coyle v. Preito, 822 S.W.2nd 596 (Tenn. App. 1991.)

Crane J. Bromberg A. Bromberg, Law of Partnership 64 (1968). Crane M. *Prescribing habits that will land you in court.* Med Econ, Vol. 67, No. 18, 17th September, 1990.

Crane M. The medication errors that get doctors sued. Med Econ, 22nd November, 1993.

Centman v. Cobb, 581 N.E. 2nd 1286 (Ind. App. 1991).

Cvetkovic D. Banovic, B. *Upravljanje rizicima od prevara sa aspekta forenzickog racunovodstva,* Zbomik radova naucne konferencije: Finansijski kriminalitet i korupcija, Institut za uporedno pravo, Institut za kriminoloska i socioloska istrazivanja, Vrsac, 2019., p. 243-258. Cvetkovic D., Micovic D., Tomic, M. *Forensic accounting and criminal work in commercial societies,* Zbornik radova Medunarodnog naucnog skupa „Dani Arcibalda Rajsa", Tom I, Krirninalisticko-policijska akademija, Beograd, 2018., p. 125 -136. Chen, A., D. Blumenthal & A. Jena. *Characteristics of Physicians Excluded from US* Medicare and State Public Insurance Programs for Fraud, Health Crimes, or Unlawful Prescribing of Controlled Substances. JAMA Network Open, 1(8), el85805. 2018, https://doi. org/10.100l/jamanetworkopen.2018.5805.

Cynthia Shea Goosen,. *How a Curbside Consult Can Land You In Court.* MedRisk Monitor, July, 1994. at l.

Ciric, J., *Nadrilekarstvo,* Pravni informator, br. 9/2006. *Comprehensive Accreditation Manual for Hospitals, Joint Commission on Accreditation of Healthcare Organizations,* Oakbrook Terrace, IL, 2001.

Coleman v. California Friends Chuck, 81 P 2d 469, 470, Cal 1938; *Schneider v. Little Company,* 151 NW, 588, Mich 1915; Pike v. Honsinger, 49 NE 760, NY 1898; "The Standard of Care, Parts I, II, and III," 225 *JAMA* No. 6, page 671, August 3, 1973; 225 *JAMA* No. 7, page 791, August 13, 1973, 225 JAMA Mo. 8, page 1027, August 20, 1973; *Adkins v. Ropp,* 14 NE 2d 727, Ind 1938.

Eisenberg H. *Patient Loyalty: you are doing something right.* Med Econ, 23rd April 1990.

David M. Harney, *Medical Malpractice,* Charlottesville VA, The Michie Company, 1993.

Dahl R. *How to get through to your patients.* Hippocrates 11 (4). Davis v. Weiskopf, III. App. 64, 439 N.E. 2nd 60, 108 III., App. 3rd 505 (1982).

Demos, MP. *The ABCs of risk management for today's practicing physician.* J Fla Med Assoc, January, 1990.

Dowling v. Lopez, 440 SE.2nd 205 (Ga. Ct. of App., Dec. 3, 1993; request rejected Feb. 22, 1994.)

Dordevic, D. *Neukazivanje lekarske pomoci,* Kazneno pravo i medicina, Tematski zbornik radova medunarodnog znacaja, Palic, 29.-30. maj 2019., Institut za kriminoloska i socioloska istrazivanja, Srbija, 2019., p.245-258.

Eremic Dodie, J., B. Laban i A. Tomic. *Forenzicka revizija - sprecavanje, otkrivanje i odgovornosti za finansijske kriminalne radje u kompanijama,* Poslovna ekonomija, br. 2., 2017 ., p. 224- 246.

Gafner RS i Launey CL. *Techniques o reducing the frequency of medical-legal lawsuits using paracommunication and neurolinguistics.* Hjuston, Medical Risk Management Inc., 1989. Dabbs M. *Take the offensive: tips for handling utilization review.* Tex Med, March, 1991.

Dahlquist CD. *The impact of technological advance on risk management.* Perspectives in Health Care Risk Management, Vol. 11, No. 4, Autumn, 1991.

Dalgo v. Landry, 424 SO.2nd 1159 (La. App. 1982)

Dashiell v. Griffith, 35 Atl 1094, Md 1896; *Capps v. Valk,* 369 P2d 238, Kans 1962.

Davison v. Mobile Infirmary, 456 So. 2nd 14 (Ala. 1984.)

Del.Code Ann. 18 6801 (&) Supp. 1984).

DeMere M. Comments of a doctor-lawyer on Chapter 54. In: Goldwyn RM, ed. *The unfavorable result in plastic surgery.* Boston: Little, Brown, 1984.

Doan v. Griffith, 402 SW 2d 855 Ky 1966; *Christy v. Saliterman,* 179 NW 2d 288, Minn 1970; *Welch v. Frisbie Memorial Hospital,* 9 A 2d 761, NH 1939.

Doctors don't discuss feed but should. Houstin Chronicle, 30th May 1992., p. 1 Oa.

Don't get sued: missed cancers. Am Med News, 25th July 1994, p. 15-16

Downer v. Veilleux, 322 A.2d 82, 87 (Me.1974); *Sprowl v. Ward,* 441 So.2d 898, 900 (Ala. 1983).

Drug administration errors in inants: don't blame individuals, fix the system. Drug and Therapeutic Perspectives 15 (9): 11/13, 2000.

Gee, J, M. Button, G. Brooks & P. Vincke, The financial cost of healthcare fraud. Portsmouth: University of Portsmouth, MacIntyre Hudson, Milton Keynes. Available at: http://eprints.port. ac.uk/3987/l/The-Financial-Cost-of-HealthcareFraud-Final-(2). pdf.

Guidelines spread, but how much impact will they have? Med Econ, 12ᵗʰ July 1993.

Federal Bureau of Investigation. Financial crimes report 2010-2011. https ://www. fbi. gov /stats-services/publications/ financial-crimesreport-2010-2011.

Federal Bureau of Investigation (FBI) 2009 Financial Crimes Report, available at: www.fbi.gov/stats-services/publications/ financialcrimesreport-2009 (accessed 8 April 2012).

Florida's grand experiment addresses practice parameters. J Florida Med Assoc, Vol. 81, No. 3, March 1994.

Fox v. Health Net of Cal., No. 219692, Ca. Super. Ct. (Riverside) (1993.)

Francoisv. Makrohisky, 67 Wis. 2nd 196,226 N.W.2nd 470 (1975.) Franklin M, Rabin R. Tort law and alternatives: cases and materials 4th ed. New York: Foundation Press, 1987.

Foundation of Research and Education American Health Information Management Association. Report on the Use of Health Information Technology to Enhance and Expand

Fought v. Solce, 821 S.W. 2nd 218,Tex.App. - Houston, 1991.

GAO, *Practitioner data bank: inormation on small medical malpractice payments.* July 1992.

Garrison v. Medical Center of Del., 581 A."nd 288 (Del. 1989.)

Gray BH. An assessment of institutional review committees in human experimentation. *Med Care* 1975; 8:318-328; Golden JS, Johnston GD. Problems of distortion in doctor-patient communications, *Psychiatry and Medicine* 1970; 50:127-148; Lee D, Bowers DG, Lynch JB. Observations on the myth of "informed consent." Plast Reconstr Surg 1976; 58:280-282.

Grunder TM. On the readability of surgical consent forms. *New Eng J Med* 1980; 302:896. Mohammed MB. Patients' understanding of written health information. *Nurs Reg* 1964; 12: 100.

Guebard v. Jabaay, 117 UI.App.3d 1, 72 III.Dec. 498, 452 N.E.2d 751 (1983) (dicta).

Gutheil et al. Malpractice prevention through the sharing of uncertainty. N Enlg. J Med 1984.; 311 (l); 49/51

Gutheil TG, Havens LL. The therapeutic alliance: contemporary meanings and confusions. *Int Rev Psychoanal* 1979; 6:467-681.

Hall v. Lundman, Scott et al., Greene County (MO) County Court, case No. 192CC2297.

Hadley, J. & J. Holahan, *"The cost of care for the uninsured: what do we spend, who pays, and what would full coverage add to medical spending?",* 2004., available at: www.kff.org/uninsured/upload/thecost-of-care-for-the-uninsured-what-do-we-spend-who-pays-andwhatwould-full-coverage-add-to-medical-spending.pdf.

Harney DM. *Medical malpractice.* The Michie Company, 1993.

Haven v. Randolph, 342 F. Supp. 538 (D.D.C. 1972.)

Hiatt HH, Barnes BA. *A study of medical injury and medical malpractice.* New Wngl. J. Med., 1989., 321: 480-484.

HMO crystallizes Albuquerque doctors' fears. Am Med News, 25th July 1994.

HMO outpatients help keep hospitals afloat. Hospitals and health networks, 5th June 1994.

How to find a doctor how really cares. McCall's, June 1994.

http://www.aahp.org/template.cfm?section=About_AAHP.

Hundley v. Martinez, 158 SE 2d 159, W Va 1967.

Hand vs Tavera 864 S.W. 2d 678 (Tex.App. - San Antonio 1993)

H. A. Thompson, *Volunteer Liability.* Tex Med, July 1991 at 58

Hall E. *The hidden dimension.* New York, Doubleday Anchor, 1966.

Helling vs Carey, 83 Wash 2nd 514, 519 P.2nd 981, 67 A L.R. 3rd 175 (1974)

Health Financing. World Health Organization, available at: http://www. who .int/ gho/health _financing/en/index. html.

Health Insurance Portability and Accountability Act 1996 (18 U.S.C., ch. 63, sec.1347.

Health Care Anti-Fraud Activities. Chicago, IL; 2005.

Heath, J. *Ethical Issues in Physician Billing Under Fee-For-Service Plans.* The Journal of Medicine and Philosophy: A Forum for Bioethics and Philosophy ofMedicine.;45(1):86-104.,2020

Hickson GB i drugi. *Factors that prompted families to file medical malpractice claims following perinatal injuries.* JAMA, 267: 10, 1359/1363.

Hoffer, E. *The American Health Care System Is Broken.* Part 7: How Can We Fix It?. The American Journal of Medicine, 132(12), 1381-1385. https://doi.org/10.1016/j.amjmed.2019.10.003.

http://www.nationalacademies.org/hmd/Reports/2012/Best-Care-at-Lower-Cost-The-Path-to- Continuously-Leaming-Health-Care-in- Arnerica.aspx.

Institute of Medicine. *Best Care at Lower Cost:* The Path to Continuously Leaming Health Care in America. Washington, DC: National Academies Press, 2012

Johnston v Sibley, 558 S.W.2nd 135, ref. n.r.e.

James v. SAD-a, 483 F.Supp. 581 N.D. (Cal. 1980.)

Jonathan M. Sykes / Managing the psychological aspects of plastic surgery patients, 2009.

Jevtic, N. Da li je nadrilekar samo prevarant, 13th November 2018, available at: https://www.pravniportal.com/da-li-je-nadrilekar-samoprevarant/, accessed: February 2022

Keddie-Holt J. *Managed care: recognzzzng and managing professional liability risks.* TMLT Reporter, Vol. 12, No. 3

Kennedy v. Parrott, 90 SE 2d 754, NC 1956; Russell v. Jackson, 221 P 2d 516, Wash 1950.

Kennedy v. Parrott, 243 N.C. 355, :-60, 90 S.E. 2d 754, 757 (1956). *Kinikin* v. Heupel, 305 n.W.2nd 589 (Minn. 1981.)

Kitto v. Gilbert, 39 colo. App. 374 570 P.2md 544 (1977.)

Kodeks medicinske etike lekarske komore Srbije, *Sluzbeni glasnik RS",* No. 104/2016.

Knezevic, S., i dr., *"Razvoj kapaciteta forenzickog racunovodstva"* grupa autora, Prevarno finansijsko izvestavanje: metode, studije slucaja i istrage, Preduzece za reviziju, racunovodstvene, finansijske i konsalting usluge „Moodys standards" d.o.o. Belgrade, 2022, Krivicni zakonik, „Sluibeni glasnik RS", br. 85/2005, 88/2005 - ispr., 107/2005 - ispr., 72/2009, 111/2009, 121/2012, 104/2013, 108/2014, 94/2016 i 35/2019.

Krstenic, J. Odnos lekara i pacijenta, 09.04.2021. available at: https://www.otvorenavratapravosudja.rs/teme/krivicno-pravo/uvod-upitanja-prava-i-zdravlja accessed: 14th February 2022

Li J, Huang KY, J. Jin & J. Shi, *A survey on statistical methods for health care fraud detection.* Health Care Manage Sci. 11 :275-287.,2008, doi: 10.1007/s10729-007-9045-4.

Lardon v. Kansas City Gas Co., lOF 2d 2634, DC Kans 1926; *Caldwell v. Missouri State Life Insurance Co.,* 230 SW 566; Ark 1921; Cameron, to use of *Cameron v. Eynon,* 3 A 2d 423, PA 1939. Laska L. *Malpractice experts: finding and using the best!* M.Lee Smith Publishers, Nashville, 1993.

Latson v. Zeiler, 250 Ca. App. 2nd 301, 58 Ca. Rprt. 436 (1967.).

Lauro v. Travelers Ins. Co., 261 So. 2nd 261, 267 (La. App. 1972.)

Lemoine v. Opste bolnice "Bunkie", 326 So.2nd 618 (La. App. 1976.)

Lidz CW, Appelbaum PA and Meisel A. *Two models of implementing informed consent.* Archives Int Med, June 1988

Loizzo v. St. Francis Hosp., 121 III.App.3d 172, 76 III Dec 677, 459 N.E.2d 314,317 (1984).

Lovenheim, Peter. *How Mediation Really Works.* Nolo Press, 1996.

Lundhal v. Rocliford Memorial Hospital Ass'n, 93 III. App. 2nd 461, 235 N.E. 2nd 674 (1968).

Lewin, K. *Field theory in social science.* New York, Harper&Row, 1951.

Likert, R. *New patterns of management.* New York, McGraw-Hill, 1960.

MacGregor, DM. *The human side of enterprise.* Njujork, McGraw-Hill, 1960.

Malpractice: Don't be a target. Louisiana Medical Insurance Company, 1990.

Mattie McDonald et. Al. Vs. Bolnice St Joseph, lawsuit No.87/38564, initiated at 152nd County Court, County Harris, Texas.

Malpractice Digest. St. Paul Fire and Marine Insurance Co. October 1984; 3.

Marvulli v. Elshire, 27 Cal.App.3d 180. 103 Cal.Rptr. 461 (1972);

Accord Thompson v. Presbyterian Hosp., Inc., 652 P2d 260 (Okla. 1982)

Matson v. Naifeh, 122 Ariz. 360, 595 P.2nd 38 (1979.)

McGeshick v. Choicair, 9 F.3rd 1229 (C.A. 7, Wisc., 15th November 1993)

McNevins v. Lowe, 40 111 209, 111 1866; Ritchey v. West, 23 111 329, 111 1860; *Barnes v. Gardner,* 9 NYS 2d 785, NY 1939. *Medical malpractice verdicts, settlements and experts.* Vol.10, No.7, 7th July 1994.

Medication Errors Symposium White Paper. Physician Insurers Association of America, Rockville, MD, 2000.

Meisel A. The "exceptions" to the informed consent doctrine: striking a balance between competing values in medical decision making.

Wisconsin Law Review 1979; 2:413-488.

Miles v. Edward O. Tabor, MD., Inc., 387 Mass. 783, 443 N.E.2d 1302 (1982); *Harvey v. Fridley Med. Center,* 315 N.W.2d 225 (Minn. 1982).

Miles v. Harris, 194 SW 839, Tex 1917.

Miller v. Dore, 154 Me. 363, 148 A.2d 692 (1959).

Mitchell v. Robinson, 334 SW 2d 11, Mo 1960.

Morse v. Moretti, 403 F 2d 564, CADC 1968.

Mull v. Emory University, 150 SE 2d 276, Ga 1966; Block.v. McVay, 126 NW 2d 808, SD 1964.

Medical science seeks a cure for doctors suffering from boorish bedside manner. Wall Street Journal, 17th March 1992

Miletic, S. i Jugovic., S. *Pravo unutrasnjih poslova,* KP A, Belgrade, 2009.

M.P.Demos, *The ABCs of Risk Management for Today's Practicing Physician,* 77 J. Fla. Med. Assoc. 37 (1990).

National Health Care Anti-Fraud Association (NHCAA *"The problem of health care fraud")* 2008, available at: www .nhcaa. org/resources/health-care-anti-fraud-resources/ theproblem- of-health-care-fraud.aspx.

Neal v Welker. 426 S.W. 2nd 476 (Ky. App. 1968).

Nealy v. U.S. Health Care HMO, 844 F.Supp. 966 (S.D.N.Y. 1994) Nikolic-Ristanovic, V., Konstantinovic-Vilic, S. *Kriminologija,* „Prometej", Belgrade, 2018.

Nikolovski, S., *Prevara i zloupotreba u zdravstvenom sistemu,* grupa autora, Prevamo finansijsko izvestavanje: metode, studije slucaja i istrage, str. 21-63, Preduzece za reviziju, racunovodstvene, finansijske i konsalting usluge „Moodys standards" d.o.o. Belgrade, 2022.

Nikolovski, S., *Prevarne radnje u zdravstvu i specificnosti njihovog identifikovanja,* grupa autora, Forenzicko racunovodstvo, istrazne radnje, ljudski faktor i prirnenjeni alati, str. 517-548,Fakultet organizacioih nauka, Belgrade, 2021.

Olson WK. *Can we ever halt America's litigation epidemic?* Med Economics, 16th September 1991.

O'Donnell WE. Who's listening? Everybody within earshot.Med Econ, 9th May 1994.

O'Riordan, WD. In-house emergencies. Emergency Medicine Risk Management, American college of Emergency Physicians, 1991. Orlikoff JE, Vanagunas AM. *Malpractice prevention and liability control for hospitals.* Chicago, America Hospital Publishing, 1998. Orlikoff JE i Vanagunas, AM. *Malpractice prevention and liability control for hospital.* Chicago, American Hospital Publishing, 1988. Paxton H. *Why doctors get sued.* Med Econ, 18th April 1989.

Parker, G. *Team players and teamwork: the new competitive business strategy.* Njujork, Jossye-Bass, 1991.

Pavlovic., B., Markovic, I., Cetkovic, P. *Pravo na zdravstvenu zastitu kroz prizmu lekarske greske,* Iustitia, Casopis udruzenja sudijskih tuzilackih pomocnika Srbije, br. 1/2016, p. 18-21.

Paripovic, V., Rajakovic, D. *Sistem zdravstvene zastite u Republici Srbiji,* Iustitia, Casopis udruzenja sudijskih i tuzilackih pomocnika Srbije, br. 1/2016, p.29-30.

Peterson vs. St. Cloud Hosp., 460 N.W. 2nd 635 (Minn. App. 1990)

Practice parameters: a physician's guide to their legal implications, Chicago, AMA, 1990.

Pravilnik o blizim uslovima i nacinu vrsenja procene zdravstvenih tehnologija ("*Sl.glasnik RS*" br. 97 /20)

Petkovic, A., Cvetkovic, D. *Interne kontrole protiv k iminalnih radnji u fimkciji pouzdanog finansijskog izvestavanja.* Revizor, Beograd, 2018., 21(82), 33-44.

Piper, C. *Healthcare fraud investigation guidebook.* Boca Raton, FL: Taylor & Francis Group, 2016

„Verdict" No. Kz. 608/03 of20.03.2003

„Verdict" Supreme Court of Serbia, Kz. I 4 78/86

"Proximate Cause, Parts I, II and III," JAMA No. 9, page 1479, Nov. 29 1971; 218 **JAMA** No. 10, page 1617, ec. 6, 1971; 218 *JAMA* No. Ll page 1761, Dec. 13,1971.

"Pure HMOs: an idea whose time may be up. Med Econ, 25th April 1994.,

Pedesky v. Bleiberg, 59 Cal Rptr 294, Cal 1967.

Perna v. Pirozzi, 92 N. J. 446, 457 A.2d 431 (1983).

Pfeffer v. Hendricks, County Ventura (Califomiaa), the Supreme Court, case No. 105645.

Phillip v. Bolnica "Good Samaritan", 65 Ohio App. 2nd 112, 416 N.E.2nd 646 (1979.)

Picket v. CIGNA Healthplan Services, Inc. No. 01/92/00803/ CV, Tex. App. - Huston [l 5t District], 17th June 1993., act rejected), 1993. WL 209858.

Practice management. Med Econ, 19th June 1989, p.43

Prather, S, Blake, RR, and Mouton, JS. *Medical risk management.* Oradell, NJ, Medical Economics Press, 1990.

Professional liability statistics for physicians practicing in Texas. Texas State Board of Medical Examiners, 2002.

Professional liability statistics for physicians practicing in Texas. Texas State Board of Medical Examiners, 1992.

Professional liability statistics for physicians practicing in Texas. Texas State Board of Medical Examiners, 1999.

Prosser WL. *The law of torts.* 4th ed. St. Paul, MN: West, 1971. *Purcellv. Zimbelman,* 18 Ariz. App. 75 500 P.2nd 335 (1972.). Randelovic, V. *Krivicno delo nadrilekarstva u teoriji i sudskoj praksi,* Pravni zivot, br. 9/2019 ., p.233-248.

Rainer vs. Grossman, 31 Cal App. 3rd 539, Ct. Of App. 2nd Dist, 11th April 1973.

Randy A. Samsone MD, Lori A. Samsone MD I Cosmetic surgery and psychological issues, Psychiatry (Edgmont), 2007.

Restatement (Second) of Agency § 220 (1958.).

Restatement§ 892A(2)(a), 892B.

Restatement (Second) of Torts 282 (1965).

Rogers v. SAD-a, 216 F.Supp. 1, 6 (S.D. Ohio 1963.)

"Res Ipsa Loquitur, Parts I-VII" 221 *JAMA* No. 5, page 537, July 31, 1972; 221 *JAMA* No. 6, page 633, Aug 7,1972; 221 *JAMA* No. 10, page 1201, Sept. 4, 1972; 221 *JAMA* No. 11, page 1329, Sept. 11, 1972; 221 *JAMA* No. 12, page 1441, Sept. 18,1972; 221 *JAMA* No. 13, page 1587, Sept. 25, 1972; 222 *JAMA* No. 1, page 121, Oct. 2, 1972.

Risk management can ease liability woes. Am Med News, 1st December 1990.

Salas vs Gamboa, 760 S.W. 2nd 838 (Tex.App.-San Antonio)

Saluja, S., A. Aggarwal & A. Mittal *Understanding the fraud theories and advancing with integrity model,* Journal of Financial Crime, 2021, ahead-of-print No. ahead-of-print. https://doi.org/10.l 108/JFC-07-2021-0163 ..)

Savic, D. *Krivicna dela protiv zdravlja ljudi,* decembar 20, 2017., available at: https://nomcentamgo.corn/krivicna-dela-protiv-zdravlja-ljudi/ accessed: 14. 02. 2022.

Savic, S. *Znacaj sudskomedicinskog vestacenja u slucajevima krivicnog dela nesavesnog pruianja lekarske pomoci,* Kazneno pravo i medicina, Tematski zbomik radova medunarodnog znacaja,, Palic, 29-30 maj 2019 ., Ins ti tut za kriminoloska i socioloska istrazivanja, Srbija, 2019., p.259-274.

Savic S. *Krivicna dela u vezi sa obavljanjem lekarske delatnosti.* Naucni casopis urgentne medicine - halo 94, Vol. 16. br. 2, 56. Beograd,2010,p. 54-65

Skalak, Golden, Clyton & Pill. *A Guide to Forensic Accounting Investigation,* New York, John Wiley and Sons Inc., 2011

Media release of the Chief Board for the Registration of Medicine (USA), 20th December, 1991.

The announcement of the Ministry of the Interior of the Republic of Serbiahttp://www.mup.gov.rs/wps/portal/sr/aktuelno/saopstenja/ d5d6e2c3- 7640-47l5-97b0-2e4dbdd892cb, accessed: 14ᵗʰ February 2022.

"Standard of Care for Specialists Parts I and II," 226 *JAMA* No. 2, page 251, October 8, 1973; 226 *JAMA* No. 3, page 395, October 15, 1973.

Strucno metodolosko upustvo za obavljanje metoda „Antiage" medicine No. 500-01-1246/2018-02 of 19.09.2018

Stojanovic, Z. *Komentar Krivicnog Zakonika Republike Srbije,* „Sluzbeni glasnik", Belgrade, 2017.

Stojanovic, Z., Delic, N. *Krivicno pravo, posebni deo,* Pravni fakultet Univerziteta u Beogradu, Pravna knjiga, Belgrade, 2013.

Simonovic, D. *Krivicna dela u srpskoj legislativi,* „Sluzbeni glasnik", 2010., p. 520.

Scheider v. Medicinskog centra Albert *Einstein,* 257 Pa. Super. 348, 349 A.2nd 1271 (1978.)

Scholoendorffv. Society of New York Hospital, 195 NE 92, NY 1914. Shrager DS. Screening and Preparing the Medical Negligence Case. trial, August 1988, p. 16-20.

Sites RL. *Emergency department closed malpractice claims: Ohio.* Perspectives in health care risk management. Vol. 10, No.2, spring, 19920. p. 17

Skelly FJ. *The payoff of informed consent.* Am Med News, 1. August 1994

Slayton v. Bruner, 276 Ark. 143,633 S.W.2nd 29 (1982.)

Sloan v. Metropolitan Health Council, 516 N.E.2nd 1104 (Ind. Ct. of App. 1987.).

Smithv. Courter, 575 S.W.2nd 199 (Mo.App. 1978.)

Sawka MP, ed. *Naic: Malpractice Claims; Final Compilation; Medical Malpractice Closed Claims;* 1975-1978. 350 Bishops Way, Brookfield WI: NAIC, 1980.

Stahlman v. Davis, 220 NW 247, Neb 1928; *Mucci v. Houghton,* 57 NW 305, Iowa 1864; *Groce v. Myers,* 29 SE 2d 553, NC 1944; McIntire, Leon L. The Action of Abandonment in Medical Malpractice Litigation. *Tulane Law Rev* 834, 1962.

Strodel RC. *Securing and using medical evidence in personal injury and health-care cases.* Prentice-Hall, 1988.

Suburban Hospital Association v. Mewhinney, 187 A 2d 671, Md 1963.

Tams v. Kotz, 530 a.2nd 1217 (D.C. App. 1987.)

The largest HMOs. Hospitals and Health Networks, 5th June 1998.

The Restatement (Second) of Agency 227 (1958).

TMLT Reporter, Vo. 9, No.2.

TMLT Reporter, Vol 10, No. 2.

To Err is Human: Building a Safer Health System. The Institute of Medicine, November 1999.

Tomes JP. *Compliance guide to electronic health records: a practical guide to legislation, codes, regulations and industry standards.* Faulker&Gray, 1994.

Toth v. Comm. Hosp. At Glen Cove, 22 N.Y.2d 255, 263 & n 2, 292 N.Y.S.2d 440, 447- 448 & n. 2,239 N.E.2d 368,373 & n. 2 (1968). *Truman v. Thomas,* 661 P 2d 902, Cal 1980.

Turner JW. *Prosecuting a medical malpractice case.* Houston Law Review, Vol. 22:535, 1985.

Tuthill E.I., *Medical staff documentation.* Tampa, FL, 1994.

Tahovic, J. *Krivicno pravo,* Posebni deo, Savremena administracija, Belgrade, 1961.

Tips to Help Prevent Medical Errors. Family Practice Management, July/August 2002

Townsend P. *Commit to quality.* New York, John Wiley&Sons, 1990

Tex Civ Prac & rem Code Ann §74.001 (Vernon 1986)

Tuthill EL. *Documentation for medical staff.* Tampa, Florida, 1994. *Vodic kroz sistem zdravstvene zastite,* available at: https :/ / www.dzblace.org.rs/wp-content/uploads/20 l 4/04NOD ICKROZ-SISTEM-ZDRA VSTVENE-ZASTITE.pdf.

The Constitution of the Republic of Serbia, *"the Official Gazette of the Republic of Serbia",* No. 98/2006.

Wilson v. Winsett, 828 S.W. 2nd 308,309.

World Health Organization, Constitution, Basic documents, Fortyfifth edition, Supplement, October 2006, Preamble.

When health plans don't want you anymore. Med Econ, 23rd May 1994, p. 138-149.

Wickline v. California, 183 Cal App 3rd 1175 (1986.).

Williams v. Good Health Plus, Inc., 743 S.W. 2nd 373 (Te Ct. App. 1987.).

Williams v. Menehan, 191 Kan. 6 379 P.2nd 292 (1963.)

The Law on Health Care, *"the Official Gazette of the Republic of Serbia"* No.25/2019.

The Law on Medical Documentation and Records in the Area ofHelth Care, *"the Official Gazette of the Republic of Serbia",* No. 123/2014, 106/2015, 105/2017 i 25/2019- dr. zakon.

The Law on the Health Care Workers' Chambers, *"the Official Gazette of the Republic of Serbia",* No. 107/2005, 99/2010 i 70/2017 - Supreme Court decision.

The Law on Medicines and Medical Devices, *"the Official Gazette of the Republic of Serbia",* No.30/2010, 107/2012, 113/2017 - other law and 105/2017 - other law.

Criminal Procedure Code, *"the Official Gazette of the Republic of Serbia",* No. 72/2011, 101/2011, 121/2012, 32/2013, 45/2013, 55/2014, 35/2019, 27/2021 - Supreme Court decision and 62/2021 - Supreme Court Decision.

The Law on the Rights of Patients, *"the Official Gazette of the Republic of Serbia",* No. 45/2013 i 25/2019 - other law.

Zarkovic, M. et al. *Kriminalistika,* VSUP, Belgrade, 1997.

Zarkovic, M., *Kriminalisticka taktika,* Kriminalisticko-policijska akademija, Belgrade, 2014.